THE COMPLETE
ILLUSTRATED
GUIDE TO

MASSAGE

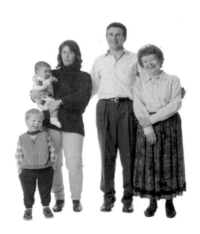

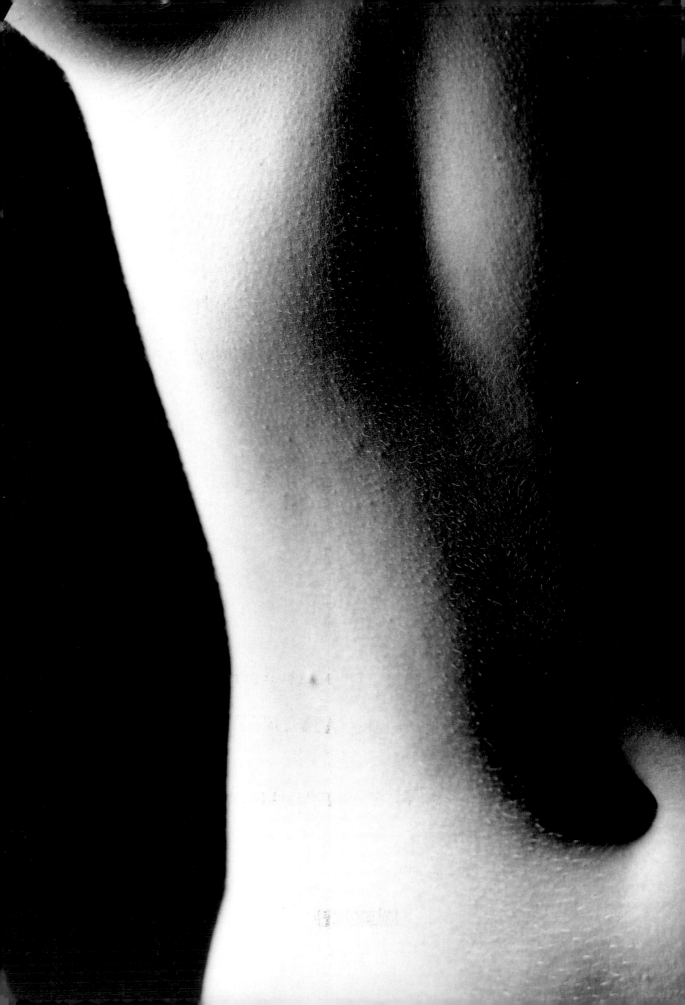

THE COMPLETE
ILLUSTRATED
GUIDE TO
MASSAGE

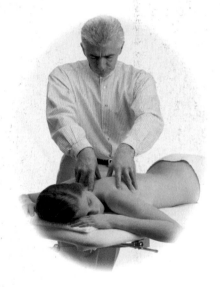

A Step-by-Step Approach
to the Healing Art of Touch

STEWART MITCHELL

ELEMENT

First published in Great Britain 1997 by
ELEMENT BOOKS LIMITED

This edition published in 2002 by Element
An imprint of HarperCollins*Publishers*
77-85 Fulham Palace Road
Hammersmith, London W6 8JB

Element™ is a trademark of HarperCollins*Publishers*

2 4 6 8 10 9 7 5 3 1

© HarperCollins*Publishers* Ltd 2002
Text © Stewart Mitchell 1997

Designed and created with The Bridgewater Book Company

Printed and bound in
Hong Kong by Printing Express

British Library Cataloguing in Publication
data available.

ISBN 0-00-713300-6

Acknowledgements

Special thanks go to:

Lewis Watson-Mitchell

Kate Faircliffe for calligraphy;
Bright Ideas, Lewes, East Sussex;
Pine Secrets, Brighton, East Sussex;
The Wilbury School, Centre for Natural Therapies,
Hove, East Sussex;
and The Plinth Company Limited, Stowmarket,
Suffolk for help with properties.

Tom Aitken, Philip Auchinvole,
Tony Bannister, Janine Bennett,
Glyn Bridgewater, Adam Carne,
Joseph Carrington-Griffin,
Rebecca Carver, Robert Chapel, Martin Comens,
Josie Coventry, Gail Downey, Nina Downey,
Rebecca Drury, Sonia Ellimann,
Carly Evans, Marcus Faithfull, Barbara Gallardo,
Cathy Glendinning, Rachel Gould, Sally Green,
Mary Harley, Paul Harley, Deborah Heath,
Julia Holden, Simon Holden, Chloe Hymas,
Janice Jones, M. Jones, Mette Lauritzen,
Carys Lecrass, Jeanne Lewington,
Denise McCullough, Norma McLean,
Kay Macmullan, Jack Martin,
Jan O'Boyle, Viv Payne, Jerry Phillips,
Bethany Pool, Sharon Rashand, Karen Riley,
Stephen Sparshatt, Rebecca Spruce,
Julie Spyropoulos, Paulette Stevens,
Robert Sullivan, Sheila Sword,
Helen Tookey, Samantha Tuffnell-Smith,
Derek Watts, Gabriel Whitelaw, Tony Wiles,
Sarah Williams, Monty Wilson, Rebecca Wilson,
and Robin Yarnton for help with photography.

The publishers wish to thank the
following for the use of pictures:
The Bridgeman Art Library: p.141T;
The Hutchison Library, p.214B;
The Royal Collection ©
Her Majesty Queen Elizabeth II: p.16;
The Science Photo Library: pp.56,
187L, 215M; Zefa: pp.14T, 19T, 33T,
38BL, 38BR, 45TL, 45ML, 49BR, 52T,
52B, 53BR, 61B, 65TR, 170R, 176T,
180T, 187BR.

CONTENTS

How to Use this Book 8
Foreword 10
Introduction 11

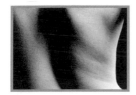

PART ONE

ALL ABOUT MASSAGE

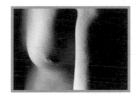

PART TWO

UNDERSTANDING YOUR BODY

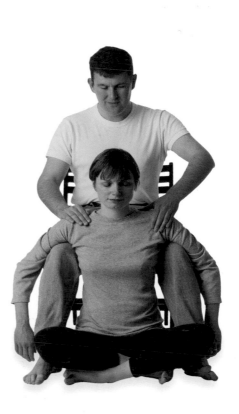

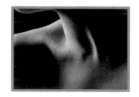

PART THREE

BASIC TECHNIQUES

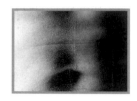

PART FOUR

MASSAGE IN PRACTICE

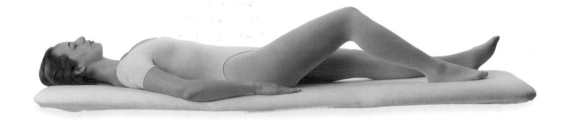

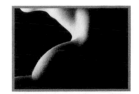

PART FIVE

SPECIAL APPROACHES AND TECHNIQUES

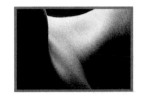

PART SIX

SPECIAL TREATMENTS

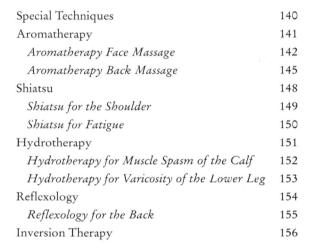

PART SEVEN

SELF-MASSAGE TREATMENTS

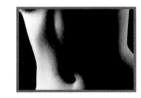

PART EIGHT

REFERENCE SECTION

HOW TO USE THIS BOOK

THE COMPLETE ILLUSTRATED *Guide to Massage* is a comprehensive introduction to the principles of therapeutic touch, written by an experienced and gifted practitioner. The book begins by placing massage within its historical, medical, and social context, as well as explaining the physiological basis of its beneficial effects. It then goes on to give a complete introduction to the massage strokes and their different effects and applications.

Part 1 gives an overview of massage as a therapy that is appropriate for all ages and that can be introduced profitably in a variety of situations – to aid recovery from illness and injury, to encourage natural bodily rhythms such as digestion and cardiovascular fitness, and to reintroduce an appreciation of touch to Western societies where people are increasingly "touch-deprived." Part 2 is a description of basic human anatomy that gives a clear picture of the body systems that benefit directly from the influence of massage.

In Part 3 the basic techniques are introduced, and Part 4 shows all the techniques in action, using clear step-by step photographs and explanatory captions. This is the core of the book and is designed both as a guide for the enthusiastic beginner and an inspiration for established practioners who want to develop new skills. Parts 5 and 6 expand on this basis to look at special approaches that embrace other complementary therapies like shiatsu and aromatherapy, and treatments for specific groups like pregnant women, babies, and the elderly. This section, like the others in the book, is illustrated with case studies drawn from practice records that show the contribution that massage can make to health in our everyday lives.

Part 7 is devoted to methods of self-massage that can be applied at home or at work so that the beneficial effects of massage can be obtained immediately. The book closes with a comprehensive reference section including useful addresses and recommended further reading.

This spread is from Part 1 of the book in which the physiological basis of massage is explained.

Main text describing the physiological background and basis of massage therapy

Box text that encourages exploration of the way your body moves

Box text giving specific information on one aspect of the body's functioning

Specially commissioned artwork

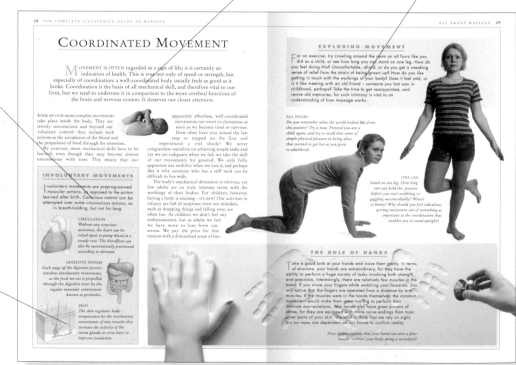

COORDINATED MOVEMENT

MOVEMENT IS OFTEN regarded as a sign of life; it is certainly an indication of health. This is true not only of speed or strength, but especially of coordination: a well-coordinated body usually feels as good as it looks. Coordination is the basis of all mechanical skill, and therefore vital to our lives, but we tend to underrate it in comparison to the more cerebral functions of the brain and nervous system. It deserves our closer attention.

SOME OF OUR most complex movements take place inside the body. They are strictly unconscious and beyond our voluntary control: they include such actions as the circulation of the blood and the propulsion of food through the intestines.

By contrast, most mechanical skills have to be learned, even though they may become almost unconscious with time. This means that our apparently effortless, well-coordinated movements can revert to clumsiness as soon as we become tired or nervous. How often have you missed the last step or tripped on the first and experienced a real shock? We never congratulate ourselves on achieving simple tasks and yet we are indignant when we fail; we take the skill of our movements for granted. We only fully appreciate our mobility when we lose it, and perhaps this is why someone who has a stiff neck can be difficult to live with.

The body's mechanical dimension is obvious, yet few adults are on truly intimate terms with the workings of their bodies. For children, however, having a body is exciting – it's new! Our activities in infancy are full of surprises; even our mistakes, such as dropping things and falling over, are often fun. As children we don't feel any embarrassment, but as adults we feel we have more to lose from our errors. We pay the price for this tension with a diminished sense of fun.

INVOLUNTARY MOVEMENTS

Involuntary movements are preprogrammed muscular actions, as opposed to the action learned after birth. Conscious control can be attempted over some unconscious actions, as in breath-holding, but not for long.

CIRCULATION
Without any conscious assistance, the heart can be relied upon to pump blood at a steady rate. The bloodflow can also be automatically prioritized according to demand.

DIGESTIVE SYSTEM
Each stage of the digestive process involves involuntary movements, as the food we eat is propelled through the digestive tract by the regular muscular contractions known as peristalsis.

SKIN
The skin regulates body temperature by the involuntary movements of tiny muscles that increase the activity of the sweat glands or erect hairs to improve insulation.

EXPLORING MOVEMENT

For an exercise, try crawling around the room on all fours like you did as a child, or see how long you can stand on one leg. How do you feel doing this? Uncomfortable, afraid, or do you get a sneaking sense of relief from the strain of being grown up? How do you like getting in touch with the workings of your body? Does it feel odd, or is it like meeting with an old friend – someone you last saw in childhood, perhaps? Take the time to get reacquainted, and revive old memories, for such intimacy is vital to an understanding of how massage works.

ALL FOURS
Do you remember what the world looked like from this posture? Try it now. Pretend you are a child again, and try to recall that sense of simple physical pleasure in being alive that seemed to get lost as you grew to adulthood.

ONE LEG
Stand on one leg. How long can you hold the posture before you start wobbling or giggling uncontrollably? What's so funny? Why should you feel ridiculous, getting enjoyment out of something as important as the coordination that enables you to stand upright?

THE ROLE OF HANDS

Take a good look at your hands and move them gently. In terms of structure, your hands are extraordinary, for they have the ability to perform a huge variety of tasks involving both strength and precision. Interestingly, there are relatively few muscles in the hand: if you move your fingers while watching your forearms, you will notice that the fingers are operated from a distance by arm muscles. If the muscles were in the hands themselves, the constant movement would make them grow too big to perform their delicate manipulations. Your hands also have great powers of sense, for they are equipped with more nerve endings than most other parts of your skin. We tend to think that we rely on sight, but our eyes are dependent on our hands to confirm reality.

How do you explain that your hand can turn a door handle without your body doing a cartwheel?

Introductory text for each group of strokes

Clear explanation of each stroke and what it is used for

This is a spread from Part 3 which introduces the massage strokes.

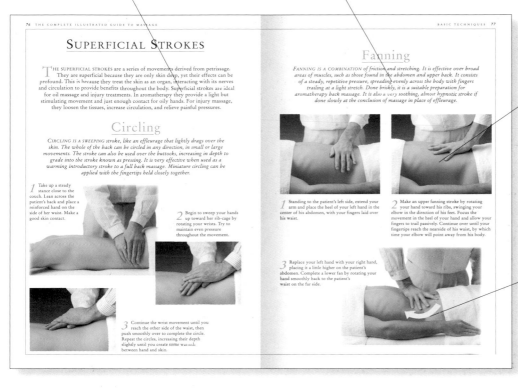

Clear photographs and captions for each step

Arrows to show direction of movement

This is an example of the case studies which show the link between massage and everyday health.

Step-by-step account of the treatment

Box copy showing how massage helped

Text explaining the background to the case study

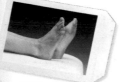

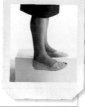

FOREWORD

I have known Stewart Mitchell for nearly twenty years. He is a gifted practitioner, and I have personal experience of his great skill in massage.

It is encouraging that he also teaches massage, because it is a largely neglected 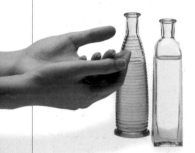 but very effective therapeutic tool. The German word for medical treatment is behandlung, which translated literally means "handling." This instructive wisdom of language hints at the healing properties of the hands, and suggests the link between massage and the "laying on of hands" in spiritual forms of healing.

Stewart has made a careful study of the manifold aspects and benefits of massage, and I am particularly pleased that he has investigated the role of massage as a self-aid and "mutual help" among family and friends. In this kind of giving the giver is twice blessed, for we hear that those who massage their friends also feel much better themselves.

The pages that follow are carefully designed to enable readers to find at a glance the aspects of massage which are of particular importance to them. I trust that this book will meet a real need, and I wish it well!

DR. GORDON LATTO MB CHB

INTRODUCTION

THIS BOOK explains how massage is almost indispensable to the restoration and maintenance of health. What exactly constitutes health, however, is open to much debate. We are often encouraged to improve our health through personal effort: by following athletic and creative pursuits or by modifying those aspects of our behavior that are commonly considered harmful. Yet such striving implies a constant struggle, which is inconsistent with a state of true happiness and wellbeing. It may be that health is not a state which must be achieved through personal effort, but an attitude toward life.

Does health equate merely to physical fitness? The frenetic pursuit of health can be confused with the fear of illness, and guilt about all our "un-healthy" habits. Asking members of an introductory massage group for a definition brought varying responses, from "curiosity," "two evacuations a day," "no pain," and "freedom from conflict." There was general agreement that expert-led health campaigns can be confusing – clouding the issue of, for example, whether to eat butter or margarine, to jog or not to jog, to keep calm at all times or express our emotions.

The concept of being medically fit was rejected by the group as a minimal definition, which tended to reduce a person to the sum of the body's parts. In contrast, a massage-inspired image of "body-mind" health emerged from the group, from discussion of our individual experience of feeling embodied. After some lively debate, a working definition of health emerged: a body which has a "mind of its own" capable of infinite expression – sensually, imaginatively, and interpersonally.

For some, health may be related to achievement of personal goals, yet many outstanding athletes and artists have not possessed perfect health. High achievers often speak of the emotional strain of success and the pressures which accompany such individuality. At the other extreme, advice to conform to safe, restrictive practices in the way we eat, drink, and proceed in life is not universally convincing, for although it is rarely disputed that too much dietary fat damages blood vessels, that smoking irritates the lungs, and that constant worrying depletes the nerves, simply avoiding these excesses does not appear to insure against ill-health.

Are there real examples of integrated body-minds who can survive success and failure, withstand occasional excess, know how to conserve and yet can "let go?" Perhaps we can be encouraged by those who, toward the end of their lives, say why they feel so satisfied. Not infrequently we hear of their spirit of enquiry and love of adventure, their enthusiasm, and willingness to take risks and become involved in life.

In this book we are going to embark on an appreciation of health, by investigating and experimenting with massage. Take a moment to realize that this will be a serious adventure: it could bring you some direct, tangible benefits, and at the same time it is likely to be a truly pleasurable experience!

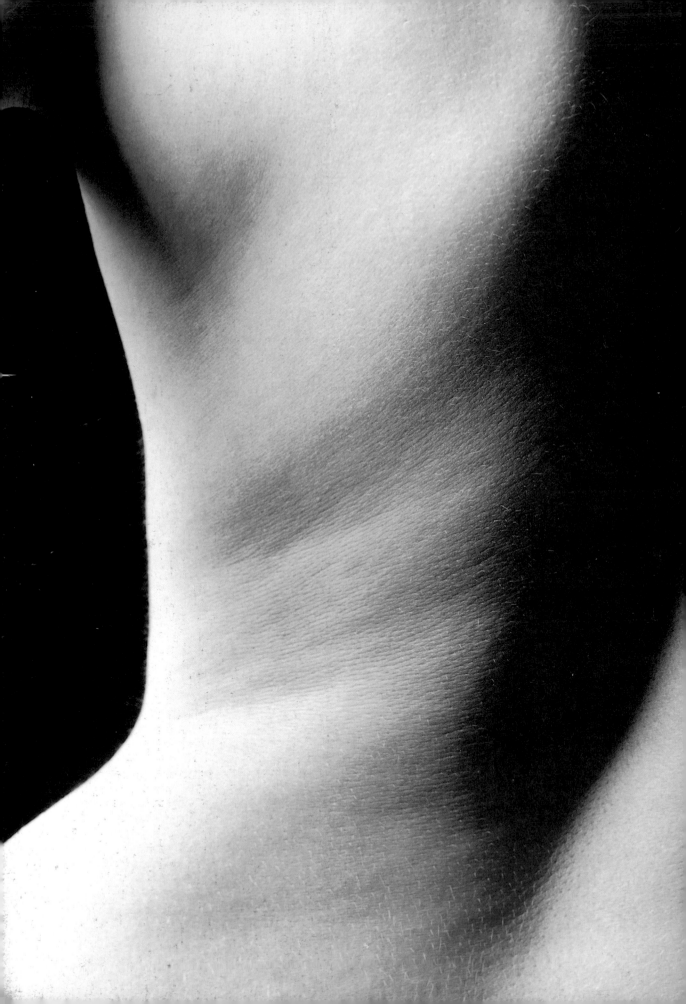

PART ONE

ORIGINS OF MASSAGE

MASSAGE IS PROBABLY one of the most popular forms of health activity today. It is used in relaxation groups and workshops, in leisure centers, and as a form of natural therapy for injury and the wear and tear of daily life. Whether performed by a trained professional or a gifted amateur, it offers the experience of touch, movement, and energy, qualities that are associated with the well-being of the whole person, and the act of giving massage has deep significance for both the giver and the receiver.

In India, kathakali dancers are traditionally treated with deep massage from the feet of their teachers.

THE PHYSICAL AND psychological benefits of massage have been recognized and valued since ancient times. Working within their limited concepts of body-function, early physicians were able to use massage very effectively in the treatment of fatigue, illness, and injury. In the fifth century B.C.E. Hippocrates described *anatripsis* – literally, "rubbing up" – as having a more favorable effect than rubbing down on the limbs, although the understanding of the blood's circulation was at that time incomplete. Esthetically, the ancient Greeks associated physical culture with the unfolding of mental and spiritual faculties, and set up massage schools in their beautifully built centers of health known as *gymnasiums*. In the Far East, performing musicians and actors have always learned massage practices as aids to their artistic development; exponents of *kathakali*, an early dance form originating in South India, are treated with deep massage from the feet of their teachers. In some societies, massage has even been used socially as an act of hospitality; in Hawaii, for example, passive movements called *lomi-lomi* are traditionally bestowed on honored guests.

In Europe, massage remained an important element of healthcare throughout the duration of the Roman Empire and is widely referred to in the literature of the era. The development of massage in the West seems to have been interrupted by the disintegration of the Roman civilization, although an unbroken tradition continued in the East. It is not until the sixteenth century, at a time when relatively sophisticated surgical techniques were being developed in France, that we hear of massage reemerging in Europe in connection with healing.

In the late nineteenth century, the demand for therapeutic massage led to the formation of societies of therapists.

DIET
The physical and emotional nourishment of massage treatment can help with irregular appetite and eating disorders.

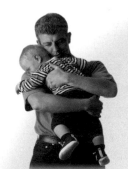

FAMILY LIFE
Simple baby massage can help instill confidence for child-rearing.

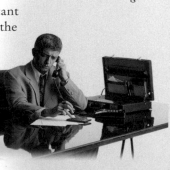

AT WORK
Some Western companies are now following Japanese custom in offering staff "massage breaks."

EVERYDAY BENEFITS OF MASSAGE
Therapeutic massage is widely recognized as being a safe and natural antidote to the stress and strain of twentieth-century living.

These societies had the objects of promoting the science of massage, organizing training, and "safeguarding the interests of the public and the profession." The desirable characteristics of a practitioner were held to be "good health, intelligence, and a high moral tone." At the time they succeeded in their aims, but later developments were to undo much of their work.

ECLIPSE AND REVIVAL

In the twentieth century, the great strides made by conventional medicine have tended to eclipse traditional therapies, even though – or perhaps because – they have been practiced for centuries. Dazzled by the achievements of science and technology, most people in the developed world all but ignored the therapeutic value of human touch until a few decades ago. Yet massage and its sister therapies are enjoying a renaissance. This can be partly explained by a return to "natural" values in reaction to the highly stressful conditions of modern life, but there is also a growing resistance to the dehumanizing aspects of modern healthcare.

OUR WONDERFUL BODIES

THE MUSCLES
Every part of the body that moves is muscular – the skin, the organs of digestion and breathing, the heart and of course the fibers of the musculo-skeletal system.

THE HEART AND CIRCULATION
Although the circulatory system contains only ten pints of blood, the powerful muscle of the heart pumps it through thousands of miles of blood vessels.

THE BONES
The 206 bones of the skeleton provide vital scaffolding for the body, yet the variety of ways they are joined together enables an extraordinary range of movements.

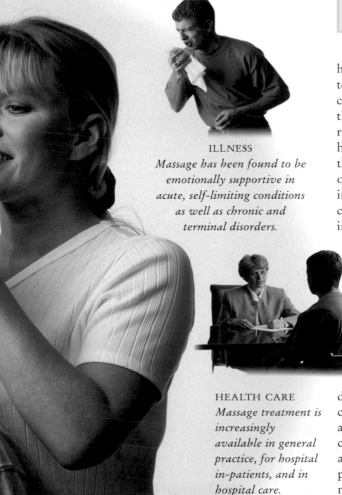

ILLNESS
Massage has been found to be emotionally supportive in acute, self-limiting conditions as well as chronic and terminal disorders.

HEALTH CARE
Massage treatment is increasingly available in general practice, for hospital in-patients, and in hospital care.

Today many people yearn for an approach to healthcare that is based, not on drugs and technology, but on the healing value of physical contact. There is nothing mystical or romantic about this idea. The human body is a physical object that responds to physical influences, and a grasp of human anatomy is central to any understanding of the role of massage. This book is partly a celebration of our wonderful anatomy: an appeal to the imagination, because anatomy *is* imagination. You can learn little about the body unless you can imagine, for example, your heart's powerful beating, the delicacy and strength of your muscles, and the balance of the bony arrangements that support you. An appreciation of the body's engineering is as vital to good massage as any psychological insight.

Massage is now firmly established as an effective therapy, yet despite growing awareness of its value, the idea of massage often meets with some resistance. Massage has been abused socially, leading to doubts about its morality, and there is still much confusion about its role in healing. Should it be seen as an alternative to conventional medicine, or a complementary therapy? How safe is it? Does it have any real physiological effects, or is it primarily psychological in value? These questions, and no doubt many more, will be clarified in the pages that follow.

TACTILE AWARENESS

Essentially, massage is a very sensitive and sensitizing form of human contact. Its medium is touch, a sense to which we humans are especially responsive. This sensitivity is developed and refined during our infancy, for during this time we are dependent on safe handling for protection and guidance in the world around us – a dependency that places great emphasis on the importance of touch. The experience of massage could

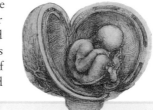

even be said to begin before birth, as the muscles of the uterus ease the baby along the birth canal. After the baby is born, its life develops into a tactile routine of holding, suckling, and caressing. This continual handling gives each of us a personal awareness of the power of human contact, and when, as adults, we experience external, given massage, the movements evoke the security of touch we experienced as infants.

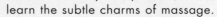

MASSAGE FROM BIRTH

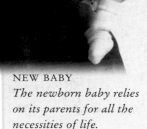

A newborn baby has little coordination or muscle tone. However, before long it is able to crawl, and the movements not only develop muscle tone but also help the baby's blood to circulate effectively. Meanwhile, the gradual acquisition of manual dexterity enables the baby to squeeze and soothe itself, and learn the subtle charms of massage.

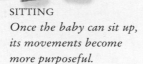

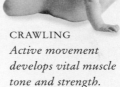

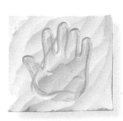

NEW BABY
The newborn baby relies on its parents for all the necessities of life.

SITTING
Once the baby can sit up, its movements become more purposeful.

CRAWLING
Active movement develops vital muscle tone and strength.

WALKING
Full coordination allows the child to walk upright.

THE REASSURING TOUCH

While a baby is in the womb, its senses are assumed to be dormant. Yet from the moment of birth it begins acquiring knowledge about sounds, focusing its gaze, recognizing smells, and, of course, exploring its world with its sense of touch. As adults we tend to rely on the more cerebral senses, such as sight and

hearing, but in infancy we are particularly dependent on the reassurance of touch. Research into child behavior shows that, given the choice between either food or comforting touch, most infants opt for touch. We can recapture that reassurance through the medium of massage.

SIGHT
Our vision is regarded as our most sophisticated sense but over a lifetime it becomes increasingly unreliable.

HEARING
Because of the importance of learning language, hearing is also highly regarded, but this sense too can decline in old age

SMELL
Our world of scent suffers from the de-odorizing tendency of modern living, but it can be rediscovered through aromatherapy.

TASTE
Subtle tastes are registered by the sense of smell, which is why food tastes strange when we suffer upper respiratory disorders.

TOUCH
People of all ages who receive massage discover that the pleasure and reassurance of touch is always available.

THE MAIN TYPES OF MASSAGE

THERE ARE MANY interpretations of massage, and each emphasizes the benefits of a particular technique or style. There are two main categories: Oriental and Western. Oriental styles tend to be stimulating, and use direct, focused pressures. Western styles are more concerned with soothing and calming the patient. The rationale for massage is quite different in each culture. Although formal anatomy is accepted in the East, practitioners there use unconventional theories to explain the interactions between the body and its "owner." So, whereas a Western therapist may speak of the liver as an organ of the body, the Eastern therapist refers to the energy that organizes the liver, and will use massage to adjust that sense of energy, rather than treat the organ in isolation.

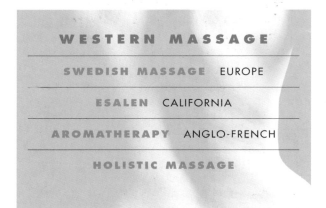

WESTERN MASSAGE

SWEDISH MASSAGE	EUROPE
ESALEN	CALIFORNIA
AROMATHERAPY	ANGLO-FRENCH
HOLISTIC MASSAGE	

PHYSIOTHERAPY

VACUUM SUCTION	EFFLEURAGE
GYRATOR	KNEADING
ULTRASOUND	PETRISSAGE
VIBRATOR	PERCUSSION

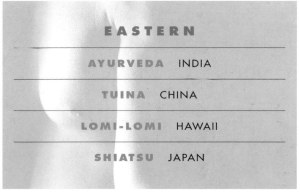

EASTERN

AYURVEDA	INDIA
TUINA	CHINA
LOMI-LOMI	HAWAII
SHIATSU	JAPAN

INTEGRATED STYLES

Both approaches are of value, and many massage therapists have integrated Eastern and Western influences into innovative styles of massage. Some of these probably reflect a reaction against technological preoccupations, since they frequently emphasize the emotional aspects of treatment. Of these approaches, reflexology is probably the most well known.

Today, one is just as likely to enjoy traditional Chinese massage in London as to receive ultrasound treatment in Beijing – such is the universal appeal of massage.

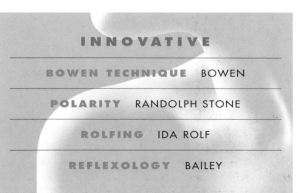

INNOVATIVE

BOWEN TECHNIQUE	BOWEN
POLARITY	RANDOLPH STONE
ROLFING	IDA ROLF
REFLEXOLOGY	BAILEY

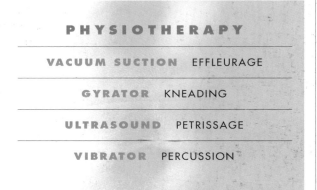

REFLEXOLOGY
The techniques employed in reflexology were practiced during the ancient Chinese civilizations, yet refined by modern Western ideas.

THE BENEFITS OF MASSAGE

THE BENEFITS OF massage are extensive. Massage can be used to help preserve
health and modify illness. It can work in conjunction with orthodox and
complementary therapies and is in itself an enjoyable and healthy activity.
As the popularity of massage increases, more opportunities are being identified
for its use – from easing the discomforts of childbirth to providing
emotional support for the prematurely aged and their near relatives.

IN INDIA, MASSAGE is considered to be
indispensable, and beneficial literally from the cradle
to the grave. In Japan, people are regularly roused by
the shiatsu practitioner who calls from house to
house asking "Shiatsu today?"; the whole family
may then each enjoy ten minutes of refreshing
treatment. Throughout the world, massage is
employed in preparation for surgery and the
manipulative adjustments of chiropractic, and it is
also used for postoperative therapy. In the United
States it is an important element of stress
management programs, and it has been found that
the act of giving simple massage
reduces stress even in the givers.

PHYSIOLOGICAL BENEFITS

The benefits of massage
as injury therapy have
always been appreciated in
sports, but in recent years
its use has developed and
expanded. Massage is now an intrinsic part of an
enlightened attitude that embraces the care as well as
the repair of athletes. Its importance as a means of
combating the stresses of competitive sports has made
it a major component of training and fitness regimes.

The value of massage as therapy for a variety of
subclinical conditions has been demonstrated by its
application to long distance air travel. Although in
some respects less arduous than in the past, modern
air journeys are nevertheless capable of producing
symptoms such as dehydration, indigestion,
stiffness, and disorientation. Massage can help with
all these, and one airline company offers inflight
therapy in which passengers receive facial, foot,
or hand massage. They are also advised on
simple de-stressing movements. Another
airline has developed a seat with
inbuilt massage technology that
intermittently stimulates passive
posture throughout the flight.

THE OLDER GENERATION
*Older people often benefit
psychologically from the intimate
touch of massage. Regular
treatment also assists the
circulation and reduces the risk
of muscle strain.*

PARENTHOOD
*Massage helps parents cope
with the worry of looking
after children, and the
strains that parenthood
can cause.*

Passengers have reported that these treatments definitely reduce the impact of jet lag, especially when combined with rest and further massage soon after arrival.

PSYCHOLOGICAL BENEFITS

It is one of the many joys of massage that its therapeutic benefits are not exclusive to professional treatment. Even at a spontaneous level, massage provides an opportunity for us to offer help to both family and friends.

It seems almost instinctive to squeeze the shoulders of a tired or anxious friend and smooth the brow of a startled child. Most people know how it feels to be under strain, and this may be our guide when giving untutored massage. For those who find it natural to extend a helping hand, it is not difficult to convert a tentative approach into a lasting, beneficial exchange for both receiver and giver. A little experience, coupled with a little knowledge about how massage works, can transform the instinctive touch into a precious gift.

Massage has been found to be a useful extension of communication between partners or colleagues when verbal and familiar patterns of relating become exhausted. Massage can

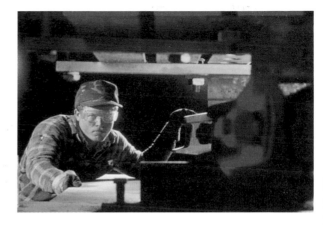

AT WORK
Most people experience stress at work, and many professions involve
physical strain of some kind. Massage provides a valuable therapy for both types of problem.

create emotional space, reducing the intensity of conflict, and provide cooling-off time without repressing the real issues. The powerful nonverbal communication of massage enables friends to address the physical burden of each other's problems without necessarily involving direct or unwanted confrontation.

ULTIMATE BENEFIT

Enjoying and appreciating the benefits of massage requires a physical receptivity and a willingness to be benefited by our bodies. Throughout history, certain religious codes of conduct have demanded restraint and control at all times and these precepts have become ingrained in our culture. Consequently, some people find their access to the pleasure of massage blocked by their own physical inhibitions. Fortunately, nature has arranged that the benefits of massage, once they have been experienced, become inviting, magnetic, and irresistible.

CHILDREN
Children often derive great pleasure from massage, and it has a useful role to play in relieving the distress of childhood illnesses. The value of massage as a means of reducing anxiety in young people is well documented.

CHILDREN AND MASSAGE

EVERY CHILD is introduced to massage within the womb by the movements of the mother's body, culminating in the contractions which propel the baby into independent life. This could be an apt analogy for a massage treatment, where the body is contained and manipulated by the practitioner's hands before being released to meet with the stresses of life. We tend to think of these stresses as an adult problem, but they have their origins in childhood.

THE BENEFITS OF INFORMAL MASSAGE can be enjoyed from the moment of birth. Babies may even experience formal massage if they are born prematurely, for studies have shown that massaging preterm infants reduces stress and shortens their stay in hospital.

As children grow older, spontaneous massage often occurs within the family when a child shows a parent where to rub after a fall. Unfortunately, this request is sometimes denied on the grounds that the child must be brave – a response that encourages the child to suppress his emotions. Such suppression can cause difficulties in later life as the individual fails to make the connection between physical and psychological symptoms.

Massage benefits children by giving a first choice, non-drug option for common aches and pains. As most childhood illnesses are self-limiting, massage offers a useful and uncomplicated method of making the child as comfortable as possible.

The effectiveness of massage on children has been measured on several occasions. One study looked at the effects of massage on a group of disturbed adolescents in an institution. For a relaxation period, half of the group were randomly assigned for massage treatment, while the other half were able to choose from video entertainment. Stress hormones sampled from the participants' blood at the end of the study showed that the massage had had a more beneficial effect.

Children with special needs respond well to massage. It provides a method of establishing contact and relieving the disorientation of a child's physical and emotional imbalance. Furthermore, since such children often require other types of treatment, massage has a useful role in developing receptivity to other therapies.

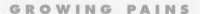

GROWING PAINS

Developing bodies can suffer discomforts, from painful feet to rounding of the shoulders. Empathetic massage can help create physical and emotional space for growth.

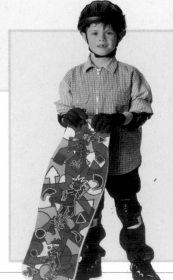

THE PLAYING FIELD

Although younger bodies are remarkably resilient and hard-wearing, minor injuries should not be ignored. Massage provides ideal conditions for effective rest and fast repair so that problems are not carried forward into later life. Of these, the most common is injury to the neck, from impact sports to falling on to the head and shoulders.

MASSAGE AND THE ELDERLY

MASSAGE IS PARTICULARLY VALUABLE as a therapy for the problems associated with growing older. Regular massage gives confidence and helps facilitate new leisure activities, as well as attending to strains and minimizing potential injury. During illness or infirmity, massage is especially supportive, relieving pressures and assisting the circulation. It also helps to relieve the sense of physical isolation that often accompanies growing older.

WE MAY SPEAK of "growing" old, but ageing is usually regarded as a process of degeneration rather than growth. Aches and pains, increasing stiffness, and reduced strength can make advancing age seem a weakened, fragile, and vulnerable state. There is an assumption that our bodies wear out through overuse, yet the fact that many active people remain healthy well into old age indicates that activity helps maintain the body.

There is certainly evidence to suggest that trying to preserve the body through non-use has the opposite effect. Analysis of the factors leading to certain age-related disorders such as osteoporosis indicates that under-use of the bones may be as destructive as overuse. In the same way, the skin is more likely to retain a healthy appearance if it is regularly subjected to friction and stretching, rather than being over-protected.

Careful massage can help provide this stimulation and enable people to maintain and extend the vitality in their lives. Obviously, people with established degenerative conditions must be treated with extra care, but, in general, older bodies can benefit from massage as direct as that given at any other age. If anything, the treatment should be more vigorous, for in clinical practice it is commonly reckoned that the older the body, the more pressure is required.

The emotional benefits of massage for later life cannot be overestimated. Loss of intimacy and a sense of isolation focus the concerns of old age, bringing apprehension about the future. Since fear tends to create rigidity, the movements of massage help break the cycle of physical and emotional strain.

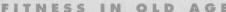

FITNESS IN OLD AGE

There may be less capacity in the older body for proper warm up procedures before activities. Regular massage provides the toning and relaxing benefits which will allow older adults to continue their active interests.

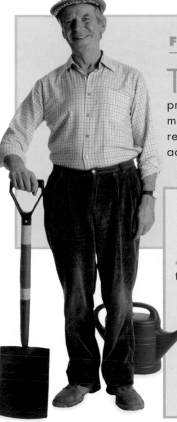

TOUCH DEFICIENCY

Although it is tempting to assume that older adults suffer from not being touched, it is equally important that they are often unable to touch another. This is borne out by studies of those who benefit from stroking pets and is confirmed by the delighted reactions of older single people giving treatments in massage workshops.

MASSAGE FOR ILLNESS

TRADITIONAL HEALTHCARE systems throughout the world recognize that massage can play an important role in treating illness. In India, for example, it is not uncommon to see children massaging the legs of their hospitalized parents. For many years, massage has been ignored by orthodox Western medicine, but, increasingly, medical practitioners have come to recognize the potential of massage therapy, especially in connection with those diseases of civilization, in which personal stress is acknowledged to be an important factor. In many such cases, orthodox treatments have achieved limited success, while holistic therapies involving massage have been of significant help.

WE RECOGNIZE ILLNESS as having two distinct aspects: "acute," which is an active or regenerative stage, and "chronic," in which degenerative processes feature. The stimulating and supportive influence of massage has much to offer in both cases, helping to alleviate acute conditions and reduce the emotional and psychological disturbance associated with chronic states.

There are circumstances in which full body massage may be inappropriate, but such circumstances rarely rule out massage entirely. Evidence from hospices where people are terminally ill suggests that, even then, a modified form of massage is entirely beneficial.

Massage is valuable during illness because of its recognition that being ill involves being disordered neurologically. The term "being ill" is another way of expressing that the body is under the dominance of the sympathetic nerves: the part of the autonomic nervous system which governs the system's response to irregularity. Sympathetic nerve activity is also associated with fear and distress, and this is why even the most simple manifestation of disease tends to be associated with emotional upset.

Extreme cases such as these are sometimes described as psychosomatic conditions, in which the fear generated and the condition provoking it fuel each other in a relentless, self-perpetuating cycle.

Massage can interrupt this cycle and relieve the distress of illness by modifying sympathetic nerve activity and encouraging the activity of the parasympathetic nerves, which have a relaxing effect. This increases the patient's tolerance of pain, which is a good indicator of recovery, enabling the patient to make a swift return to full health.

ILLNESS AS "DIS-EASE"

Being ill usually involves feeling uncomfortable, and easing that discomfort is part of the recovery process. This is where massage can help. It relieves the discomfort of the inflammatory processes that accompany illness by diverting the blood supply, an effect that is well illustrated by rubbing your cold feet during a headache. Since there is only a limited amount of blood circulating in your system, stimulation of one part of the body will draw blood impetus toward that part; in consequence, any congested areas will be relieved of pressure.

ILLNESS AS "DIS-ORDER"

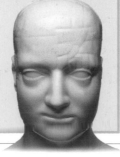

The attempt to categorize illnesses as belonging to either the body or the mind gave rise to the separate disciplines of physical and psychiatric medicine, but this is alien to massage. Organic symptoms are almost always accompanied by psychological distress, and emotional problems are rarely without physical manifestations.

MASSAGE FOR INJURY

THE INFLUENCE OF massage on the circulation is very helpful in alleviating pain after accidents and injuries. In the case of serious injury, the pain can be greater during the recovery stage than immediately after the accident, and is often associated with the return of functioning. Vigorously massaging the opposite limb to the injured one, or the lower limbs in cases of upper body injury, alleviates pressure without compromising the healing processes.

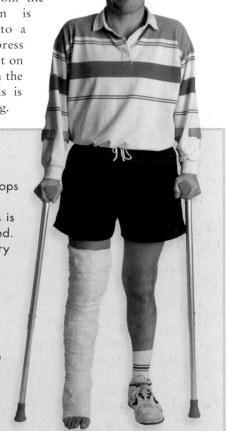

AN INJURY CAUSES discontinuity of the tissue, interrupting normal functioning. It is accompanied by pain, swelling, and inflammation. Pain draws conscious awareness to the site of the injury so that irritating movement is discouraged. The increased circulation to the injured tissue is responsible for the swelling, which also helps immobilize the damaged area. Inflammation involves a rise in local temperature that helps destroy debris within the injury. Appropriate massage treatment helps modify these responses so that injuries are easier to bear and quicker to heal.

The blood that is attracted to an injury is thicker than usual because of the increase in white cell activity. The lymphatic system is also mobilized to supply a watery disinfectant that protects the body from any external contamination. It is unwise to reduce the resulting swelling artificially since it contains healing ingredients. Raising the injured part higher than the heart usually makes the congested state much more tolerable; meanwhile the gentle strokes of massage, above and below the injury, are helpful in maintaining an effective drainage.

The inflammatory response is necessary to help dispose of disintegrating body tissue. It is an uncomfortable experience, however, and the most obvious, effective way to minimize this discomfort is through the use of cooling hydrotherapy. The heat from the inflammation is transferred to a cool compress and the effect on the nerves in the blood vessels is very soothing.

MASSAGE AND RECOVERY

It is tempting to assume that an injury has recovered when it stops being painful. In fact, the most reliable indicator is swelling. Premature use of an injured part will increase swelling, and this is evidence that the unfinished healing processes are being irritated. Continued use of the injured part will simply reverse the recovery process, a fact that is soon made evident by returning pain.

Although an injured person may feel the need to get back to normal functioning as soon as possible, rest and poise are as important as specific exercise. The idea that an injured person must exercise energetically to ensure recovery is no more valid than the theory that he should overeat to maintain his strength. Exercise programs that require an almost heroic application are based on fear and are unnecessary. The passive, active, and resistive exercises which complete a full body massage are sufficient to build the flexibility, strength, and coordination required during the recovery stage.

THE EFFECTS OF MASSAGE

WHEN YOU HAVE had some experience of the methods, both you and your partner will begin to realize why massage has such a deserved reputation as a therapy. Therapeutic massage is effective because it is pro-biotic: it assists the normal functioning of the body and provides an emotional safety valve to reduce the anxiety that health problems can provoke. The permission we give others to massage us is not given lightly, however, and it is the establishment of trust and cooperation that allows the strokes of massage to relieve both physical and emotional discomfort.

THE BENEFICIAL EFFECTS of massage begin with its influence on the muscular tissues of the body. Skillful manipulation of the muscles assists the circulation of the blood and lymphatic fluid, stimulates the organs of digestion, and improves the performance of the lungs and skin. As the muscles improve in tone, so do the nerves that supply them, right back to the spinal cord and the brain.

The extent to which massage can influence the rhythmic functioning of the body makes it particularly effective in helping to treat the disorders that are caused by the complexities of modern life. Cardiovascular diseases, for example, are strongly associated with such personal and environmental factors, and massage has proved itself a valuable therapy, even in the most advanced stages of heart disease. It is regularly employed as part of the rehabilitation process after cardiac arrest.

Most people find massage increases awareness of the body, raising their levels of energy and leading to an enhanced feeling of well-being. Massage treatment achieves this through gentle, persistent focusing on the whole person, to provide a refreshing perspective on long-standing problems – regardless of whether these are physically based or psychologically induced.

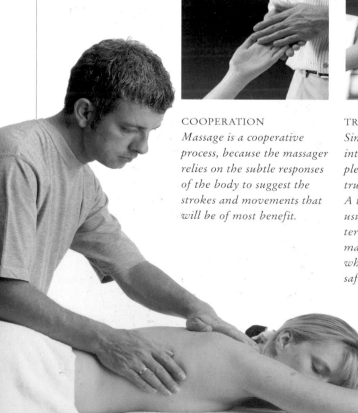

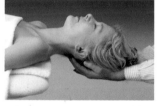

COOPERATION
Massage is a cooperative process, because the massager relies on the subtle responses of the body to suggest the strokes and movements that will be of most benefit.

TRUST
Since massage is both an intimate and potentially pleasurable therapy, shared trust is of vital importance. A trusting relationship is usually seen in psychological terms, but it is established in massage by physical contact, which makes the body feel safe, and safe to be with.

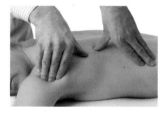

TOUCH
It is paradoxical that while the skin functions as a physical barrier to infection, it also acts as a sensitive receptor of touch: the sensation by which we appreciate the strokes of massage. Yet permitting even the touch of massage to penetrate the skin's defenses can seem like an intrusion. The removal of this psychological barrier is essential to the effectiveness of massage.

MEASURABLE BENEFITS OF MASSAGE

THE NERVOUS SYSTEM
Nerves are great communicators, and they appreciate the conversations that take place during massage. Painful nerves are soothed by the monotone of smooth stroking, while tired nerves are helped to rest by the lullabies of rhythmic squeezing. Massage can reassure "trapped nerves;" they are not really trapped, but just feel that way.

THE EMOTIONS
Unexpressed emotion is often contained in hypertense muscles, and in this way emotions can be directly addressed by massage. The shoulder muscles are also commonly recognized as reservoirs of dysfunctional tension. The movements of massage provide a counterpressure that tends to dissipate tension, freeing it to be converted into energy.

THE LUNGS
Massage movements eliminate tension in the chest, shoulders, and abdomen to permit full breathing. Percussion strokes, especially at the sides of the chest, help clear the airways. Respiratory massage also helps with emotional readjustment.

THE HEART
The heart is really a distended blood vessel that generates and sustains the high pressures needed to circulate the blood through the body, so the direct influence of massage on the arteries and veins is welcome. Nervous pressure in the heart is reduced by simple neck massage, which steadies the heartbeat.

DIGESTION
The most profound effect of massage on the digestive system is to relieve the stress responses that impede digestion. Digestive massage is a good self-treatment, which begins with tongue and gums in the morning and is completed by lower abdomen massage just before sleep. Stroking toward the digestive organs stimulates peristalsis, the spontaneous massage action of the intestines.

THE MUSCLES
Muscles are toned by massage, which stimulates their reflexes and redistributes their tension. This enables them to contract efficiently and in coordination to give grace to our movements. The warming strokes and cooling stretches of massage are good preparations for activity and rest.

PLEASURE
Massage becomes pleasurable as the body accepts that the strokes and pressures are not harmful, and such agreeable sensations have long been recognized as an effective way of combating pain. Ultimately, the pleasure of massage is such that, for the practitioner, learning how to terminate a massage is as important as learning how to perform it.

INJURIES
After injury, gentle whole-body massage conveys reassurance. Smooth stroking reduces pain by relieving the congestion of the healing process. Later, friction massage near the injury site speeds repair by stimulating the circulation.

MASSAGE FOR LIFE

THERE IS NOTHING alien about the rhythms of massage. Rhythmic movements can be observed throughout nature, from the ebb and flow of the tides to the barely detectable pulsations of plants, and similar rhythms are intrinsic to the workings of the human body. Your body is constantly massaging itself as it moves, and this automatic massage is vital to health. Applied massage simply complements the natural rhythms of life, and is particularly valuable when those rhythms have been inhibited by inactivity.

BODY DESIGN

The principles of massage are largely inspired by the natural movements of the body. The following are three examples of the way your body looks after itself, and as you become aware of them you will appreciate the possible benefits of massage.

DIAPHRAGM

The diaphragm muscle at the base of your chest compresses and releases your digestive organs with each breath. Your stomach and liver are the main beneficiaries of this action, since it ensures efficient blood supply.

MUSCLES

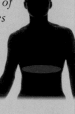

The heart pumps blood to the extremities of your body, but the return flow is propelled by the limb muscles. The muscle contractions squeeze the veins to shunt the blood back toward the heart and lungs, often against the force of gravity. If this squeezing does not occur, your limbs feel heavy and become numbed.

WALKING

Since we are basically four-legged creatures who have taken to standing upright, we need to swing our arms as we walk. Without this complementary walking action, the movement initiated by the lower back is blocked at the shoulders, creating tension; walking then becomes far more strenuous.

YOUR BODY'S SELF-MASSAGE system is normally reliable, but it can become inhibited and body functions can suffer dramatically. The effect of gravity alone is a constant challenge to your circulation, but the absence of physical stimulus and the monotony of routine are more powerful undermining factors.

The self-massaging internal rhythms of your body are also less effective if you try to live outside your natural body clock by overextending yourself beyond physical warning signals, such as pain or dizziness. It is at such times that people need applied massage. This can be illustrated by two examples from everyday life.

When you are unwell or tired, many of your natural body movements become depressed. You may notice that if you have to sit still over a long period, your lower legs seem to fill up. If you've slipped your shoes off, as you might do on a long journey, they will probably feel too small when you try to put them back on. This is because the natural massaging movements of your legs have been inhibited by sitting still, and the effect of gravity is slowing the circulation in your feet. Unremedied, this may induce headache or drowsiness. A few minutes devoted to the simple massage movements of wringing and stroking will soon correct the situation, and you will feel the benefit throughout your body.

You may have experienced local stiffening after a collision or fall, or perhaps after an unpleasant emotional exchange. Muscles and joints that normally glide effortlessly under your skin become painfully reluctant, and you move cautiously because, after even the mildest trauma, your body wants to play safe for a while. Eventually, you may recover a sense of physical and mental composure, but very often you are too busy or exhausted to make a quick recovery. Massage intervention can be valuable, since it not only eases and loosens the tissues, but also creates a reassuring atmosphere that reduces tension.

DEPRESSED BODY MOVEMENTS

When the body is tired or unwell it tends to collapse, instinctively asking to be laid down somewhere undemanding. Much of the blood supply gets diverted deep into recuperative organs such as the kidneys or liver, so trying to sit upright using drained muscle power leads to strain.

HEADACHE
Keeping the neck in a rigid posture, usually forward of center, increases tension toward the back of the skull. This is where the neck muscles have to work hard to hold the head up. Excessive tension in these muscles leads to a classic headache, because it inhibits the circulation from the head – the eyes in particular – during periods of extended concentration.

LOWER LEGS FILL UP
Extended periods of sitting down inhibit the circulation from the legs because the blood vessels are constricted by the fixed flexion at the pelvis. In time they also come under pressure from a "collapsing" upper body. The lower leg makes another flexion at the knee, an effect made worse by leg-crossing. The legs seem to fill up uncomfortably.

SWOLLEN ANKLES
The ankles contain more bones than any other joints. When maltreated by being kept immobile and at the mercy of gravity, they naturally object by swelling up. This is also a defensive mechanism, since the accumulated fluid discourages the ankles from being moved too quickly after a long period of inactivity, which could cause injury.

LOCALIZED STIFFENING

A minor injury such as a fall, or even an argument, can lead to a localized, painful stiffening of the muscles and joints. This is one of the body's natural defense responses.

STIFFENING
We stiffen in response to unexpected experiences. Stiffening has the overall effect of providing time to process a response and generate flexibility. If the experience was a physical confrontation, you can prepare in anticipation of the next time. If the experience was emotional, you can rehearse a response mentally.

BALANCE
Balance is a product of forces that work antagonistically to create composure. Good balance relies on energy and awareness, for, without these, any one force has the capacity to dominate the others.

PAIN
Pain is essentially a protective reaction, since it alerts the body to a problem and often prevents actions that could cause further damage. Pain can indicate injury, but it can also hint at unrecognized tiredness. Pain can suggest alteration, modification, or cancellation.

MUSCLE TENSION
Physical or emotional trauma increases muscle tone and initially puts the body on alert. Where there is physical damage, tense muscles provide a restraining influence to prevent further damage.

COORDINATED MOVEMENT

MOVEMENT IS OFTEN regarded as a sign of life; it is certainly an indication of health. This is true not only of speed or strength, but especially of coordination: a well-coordinated body usually feels as good as it looks. Coordination is the basis of all mechanical skill, and therefore vital to our lives, but we tend to underrate it in comparison to the more cerebral functions of the brain and nervous system. It deserves our closer attention.

SOME OF OUR most complex movements take place inside the body. They are strictly unconscious and beyond our voluntary control: they include such actions as the circulation of the blood and the propulsion of food through the intestines.

By contrast, most mechanical skills have to be learned, even though they may become almost unconscious with time. This means that our apparently effortless, well-coordinated movements can revert to clumsiness as soon as we become tired or nervous. How often have you missed the last step or tripped on the first and experienced a real shock? We never congratulate ourselves on achieving simple tasks and yet we are indignant when we fail; we take the skill of our movements for granted. We only fully appreciate our mobility when we lose it, and perhaps this is why someone who has a stiff neck can be difficult to live with.

The body's mechanical dimension is obvious, yet few adults are on truly intimate terms with the workings of their bodies. For children, however, having a body is exciting – it's new! Our activities in infancy are full of surprises; even our mistakes, such as dropping things and falling over, are often fun. As children we don't feel any embarrassment, but as adults we feel we have more to lose from our errors. We pay the price for this tension with a diminished sense of fun.

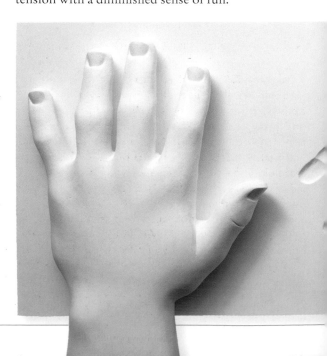

INVOLUNTARY MOVEMENTS

Involuntary movements are preprogrammed muscular actions, as opposed to the action learned after birth. Conscious control can be attempted over some unconscious actions, as in breath-holding, but not for long.

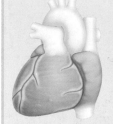

CIRCULATION
Without any conscious assistance, the heart can be relied upon to pump blood at a steady rate. The bloodflow can also be automatically prioritized according to demand.

DIGESTIVE SYSTEM
Each stage of the digestive process involves involuntary movements, as the food we eat is propelled through the digestive tract by the regular muscular contractions known as peristalsis.

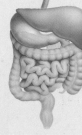

SKIN
The skin regulates body temperature by the involuntary movements of tiny muscles that increase the activity of the sweat glands or erect hairs to improve insulation.

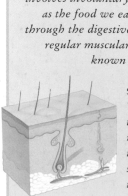

EXPLORING MOVEMENT

For an exercise, try crawling around the room on all fours like you did as a child, or see how long you can stand on one leg. How do you feel doing this? Uncomfortable, afraid, or do you get a sneaking sense of relief from the strain of being grown up? How do you like getting in touch with the workings of your body? Does it feel odd, or is it like meeting with an old friend – someone you last saw in childhood, perhaps? Take the time to get reacquainted, and revive old memories, for such intimacy is vital to an understanding of how massage works.

ALL FOURS
Do you remember what the world looked like from this posture? Try it now. Pretend you are a child again, and try to recall that sense of simple physical pleasure in being alive that seemed to get lost as you grew to adulthood.

ONE LEG
Stand on one leg. How long can you hold the posture before you start wobbling or giggling uncontrollably? What's so funny? Why should you feel ridiculous, getting enjoyment out of something as important as the coordination that enables you to stand upright?

THE ROLE OF HANDS

Take a good look at your hands and move them gently. In terms of structure, your hands are extraordinary, for they have the ability to perform a huge variety of tasks involving both strength and precision. Interestingly, there are relatively few muscles in the hand: if you move your fingers while watching your forearms, you will notice that the fingers are operated from a distance by arm muscles. If the muscles were in the hands themselves, the constant movement would make them grow too big to perform their delicate manipulations. Your hands also have great powers of sense, for they are equipped with more nerve endings than most other parts of your skin. We tend to think that we rely on sight, but our eyes are dependent on our hands to confirm reality.

How do you explain that your hand can turn a door handle without your body doing a cartwheel?

CASE STUDY 1

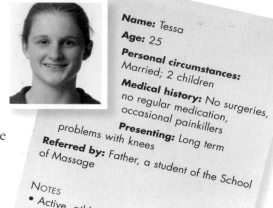

Name: Tessa
Age: 25
Personal circumstances: Married; 2 children
Medical history: No surgeries, no regular medication, occasional painkillers
Presenting: Long term problems with knees
Referred by: Father, a student of the School of Massage

NOTES
• Active, athletic physique; aims to keep fit
• Positive personality

THIS CASE STUDY demonstrates the advantage of looking at mechanical problems from the wider perspective of massage therapy. Massage therapists are aware that one part of the body rarely suffers in isolation. The body develops as an integrated system, and this means that pain is sometimes referred from one area of the body to another and that function of a damaged area is often maintained by indirect compensation of related structures.

SYMPTOMS	ASSESSMENT	TREATMENT
• Chronic pain in knees over a long period • No response to drug treatment or physiotherapy • Anxiety about possible surgery or loss of mobility	• Knees basically normal, but with hyper-extension • Deeply hollowed back • Weight shifted toward front of feet	• Massage to stretch the back muscle and relieve spine tension • Massage to reduce tension in the knees and improve muscular control • Advice on how to stretch the back muscles and rest the knees

IN TESSA'S CASE, her body was attempting to relieve a complex tension by transferring it to a more obvious site where it could be released. This had been diagnosed as a local problem and became the focus of pathological interpretation.

FIRST TREATMENT

Tessa described how she had experienced very painful knees since her teens. She had been given drug treatment and physiotherapy, but with no beneficial effects. As someone who had performed gymnastics at a high level, and who had never experienced any leg injury, she was confused about the cause of her pain. She was also trying to come to terms with an offer of surgery, which her specialist recommended unless she was to "become seriously debilitated by her 30th birthday."

On examination in the standing position, Tessa's knees appeared normal, although they displayed some hyperextension or "swayback" posture. In profile, the lower back was deeply hollowed and the weight of the body was shifting towards the front of the feet.

Simple massage was given to the knees. This caused no pain, but there was tightness in the muscles at the front of the thighs. Treatment to the lower back revealed some tenderness, and mild pressure caused the back muscles to contract. It was apparent to the patient that, in the horizontal position, greater problems existed in the lower back than in the knees, and it was explained that the knees can be influenced by the tensions placed upon them from above. The back muscles were massaged slowly and deeply and given firm stretching. Tessa was also advised on how to gently stretch her back muscles at home and rest her legs by placing a pillow under the knees, with feet raised.

SECOND TREATMENT

Tessa had experienced some pain-free days after the first treatment. She found the home exercises restful, and she felt more optimistic about the future. She had begun to notice that sensations of unease originated in her back before she was conscious of pain in her knees.

Further treatment was given to the back muscles, to continue the lengthening process and relieve pressure on the spine. The front of each leg was massaged to help condition the muscle tone by discouraging tension. The muscles on the back of the thighs were stimulated to exert a controlling influence on the knee's forward movement.

After this the patient felt confident enough to consider that her basic fitness, together with regular massage sessions, would overcome her problem. She was given a program of back and awareness exercises to maintain progress, and was encouraged to rest as much as she exercised.

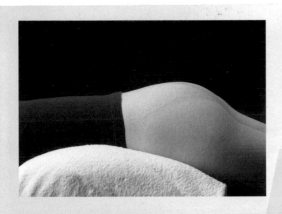

SELF-HELP: PAIN RELIEF
Lying over a pillow placed under the abdomen or pelvis will reduce pressure in the lumbar area. This will help relieve pain from the spine, lower abdomen, and legs. A second pillow may be positioned under the feet.

SELF-HELP: REST THE LEGS
Placing a pillow under the knees when resting relieves tension. Raise the legs and flex the knees slightly so that the leg muscles are just stretching.

SELF-HELP: KNEES TO CHEST
Standing close to a table, step up and place the left foot flat. By bending the supporting leg, the lower back has a controlled stretch on the left side. Aim to just touch the buttock on to the table, keeping both feet flat. Recover slowly and repeat the stretch to the other side of the back.

SIGN OF LORDOSIS
Hollow back or lordosis is easily observed in profile if an imaginary plumbline is dropped from the center of the ear; ideally, the line should pass through the shoulder, hip, and ankle.

HOW DID MASSAGE HELP?

- The positive assessment after examination of the knees and the information that healthy, active people rarely become seriously disabled was very reassuring. It allowed the massage treatment to produce beneficial effects immediately.
- By identifying the lower back as the primary source of the problem in the knees, further deterioration was prevented.
- Massage helped Tessa to understand how tension in her body could be related to other stresses, and gave her confidence in her ability to overcome the negative image of her problem.

CASE STUDY 2

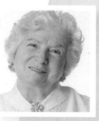

THIS CASE STUDY illustrates how massage helped solve a problem by bringing about a resolution of emotional conflict. The problem had previously been treated as a purely physical condition, and it is often difficult for people to get suitable treatment for health problems because they themselves are confused about the real cause of their difficulty. However, since for many people the greatest influences on their lives are other people, relationships should always be considered as possible factors.

Name: Elizabeth
Age: 73
Personal circumstances: Single, living in nursing home
Medical history: Minor surgeries, no medication, no serious medical history
Presenting: Dizziness
Referred by: Existing patient

NOTES
• Not very active, overweight (long-term), sleeping poorly, appetite good, vegetarian
• Cheerful on the surface but obviously distressed
• Recently diagnosed with high blood pressure. Nursing home told to put her on a diet, but no change in blood pressure after three weeks.

SYMPTOMS	ASSESSMENT	TREATMENT
• Dizzy spells, at least once daily • Continued high blood pressure • Anxiety	• Neck and shoulders very tight • No contraindication to massage • General health and fitness reasonable for age	• Shoulder and neck massage • Advice on self-massage and breathing exercises • Dialogue with practitioner

FIRST TREATMENT

During the first consultation, Elizabeth described her feeling of dizziness, which affected her at least once daily. She was adamant that her new diet regime was not helpful to her blood pressure condition, since she liked eating. The diet was producing anxiety, making her want to eat even more.

On examination, her neck and shoulders were found to be very tight, a symptom consistent with anxiety. Light massage was given in the seated position, with regard to elevated blood pressure. During the treatment the patient began to speak of emotional strain associated with the reappearance of an old acquaintance who had moved into a neighboring room in the nursing home. Events dating to many

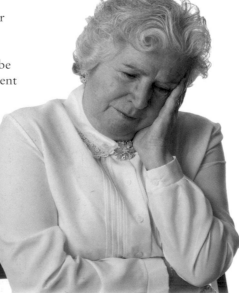

years before made this person's presence disturbing. Elizabeth felt unable to express this.

It was explained that tense shoulders and emotional upset are sometimes directly connected, and the first treatment ended with some advice on self-massage of the neck and deep breathing.

SECOND TREATMENT

When the patient came for her second treatment there was no change in her medical condition, and more tension in her neck and shoulders. During this session the patient became visibly distressed and spoke of the background to the emotional upset. Her shoulders became much more massageable, although distress continued throughout the treatment.

THIRD TREATMENT

On her third visit Elizabeth was much brighter. Her doctor had recorded a slight lowering of blood pressure, and she was eating more.

The shoulder and neck massage continued, and during treatment she described how she had approached her former acquaintance and shared her feelings. She felt a great release within after attempting to air their differences with her neighbor, and by the end of the massage session she was happy to return to her familiar routine.

HOW DID MASSAGE HELP?

• Sometimes a medical diagnosis is a welcome distraction from a problem, but in this case it only emphasized an aspect of the problem, and in a punitive way. Massage highlighted another focus of pressure, in the neck and shoulders, to which the patient could connect emotionally.

• The treatment of the neck and shoulders eased the circulation between the arms and chest, which tends to become restricted with anxiety. Nervous controls shared by the arms and chest were also influenced to induce deeper breathing, which in itself helps relieve pressure.

• The treatment enabled Elizabeth to use the supportive atmosphere of the massage session to express herself. This is not the same as a response in conventional psychotherapy. Her dialogue with the practitioner was able to move between the tactile and verbal according to her feelings: when words failed, focus returned to the muscles; when tension was greatest, words came.

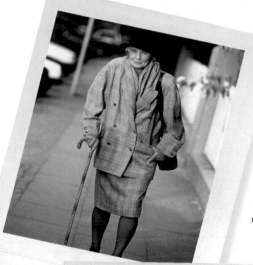

SELF-HELP: KEEP ACTIVE
Increasing the movement of the whole body is the most appropriate physical response to increased blood pressure. Several short walks taken throughout the day are preferable to longer trips, which can become tiring on the return journey.

SELF-HELP: HEAT
Using a hot towel to apply moderate heat to the back of the neck is comforting and helps unlock the muscles. As pressure is released, feelings of vulnerability give way to more positive attitudes.

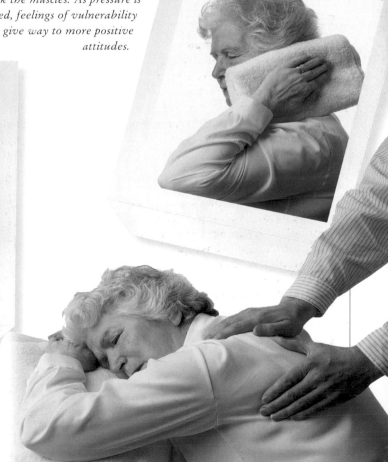

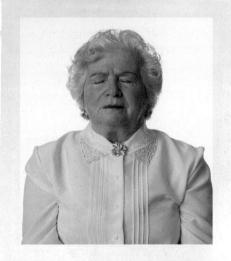

SELF-HELP: PRACTICE DEEP BREATHING
Breathing deeply is a positive statement and helps clear confusion. Improved posture of the chest also raises the spirits, enhances confidence, and increases the capacity to bear stress.

FIT FOR MASSAGE: POSTURE

THE CONCEPT OF fitness implies a type of well-being, which is about active participation in life coupled with an ability to withstand the pressures involved in an active lifestyle. Some people appear to be born with a greater dynamism than others, and we think of them as having strong constitutions. This is another way of saying that such people have the stamina provided by robust cardiovascular systems, which not only allows them to be more active, but also protects them from the stresses and strains of life.

CARDIOVASCULAR FITNESS consists of efficient breathing and blood circulation and a balanced posture. It is achieved by the use of the body in free movement, which encourages communication between the heart, muscles, and nervous system. The reward for this is to be able to move about efficiently, economizing on effort and avoiding overexertion. Fitness regimes may be necessary to raise the body to a desirable level of cardiovascular efficiency, but, in theory, once achieved it should be possible to maintain it simply by practicing the freedom of movement it provides.

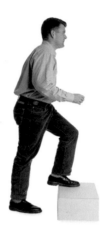

ADULT DECLINE

Most of us develop healthy freedom of movement during childhood, but as we grow, the restrictions of adult life, often self-imposed, begin to undermine our fitness. A sedentary occupation, dependence on the car, and passive recreation are rapidly becoming the norm, both for adults and, increasingly, for children. This results in life becoming a predominantly neurological experience that is not complemented by physical expression, and the consequences for fitness are entirely negative. The tension in our systems contributes toward the hypertension – high blood pressure – now said to affect 25 percent of males in the United States and the U.K. In some industrial countries, cardio-vascular unfitness can be held responsible for the majority of fatal diseases.

CYCLES OF TENSION

Before chronic health problems become fully manifest, our posture often provides ample evidence of tension. When low-level stresses are not resolved satisfactorily, we are inclined to distort our bodies. In parallel situations, other animals attempt to grow in size by arching their backs high, widening their chests or rearing onto their hind legs. A human being, by contrast, is apt to make himself smaller by retracting his neck, tightening his arms against his chest, or wriggling his pelvis around to one side. These defensive actions provide time to devise an appropriate way of dealing with the problem. However, if the difficulty concerns an overbearing employer, a family difficulty, or an emotional relationship that cannot be immediately solved, the failure to settle the matter simply results in more stress, creating a vicious cycle. Attempting to come to terms with intractable problems leads to muscle tension over long periods. The danger, of course, is that this unexpressed tension becomes a major problem in itself, producing neurological symptoms often much more complicated than those that might have resulted from submission to the original difficulty. There is a further difficulty in that prolonged tension causes the body to communicate inappropriately. People who are jumpy are liable to find that even their simplest communications are misunderstood.

THE ROLE OF MASSAGE

Massage can address this state of tension directly, and therefore help deal with the underlying emotional problems. It may take time, however, because this over-tensing represents an investment in self-protection and can become habitual. Fortunately, massage is able to confront tension without seeking to remove it prematurely. It achieves this through patient, reassuring touch. Massage therapy recognizes the reality of problems, but helps to put them into perspective. It reaffirms human contact, which is sufficient to break unhelpful cycles of tension and free the muscles to respond to life's pressures creatively and energetically.

THE ORIGINS OF FAULTY POSTURE

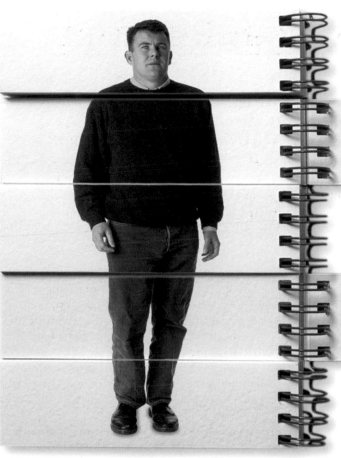

TIGHTENING THE ARMS *against the chest restricts breathing, and therefore the movement that might give away a hiding place. This posture is adopted in the hope that troubles will pass by, but restricted breathing causes its own problems.*

WRIGGLING THE PELVIS *around to one side is a gesture of partial advance toward or withdrawal from a problem, because the feet have not carried through the decision. It produces a backache that suggests conflict and indecision.*

A RETRACTED NECK *is an instinctive response to perceived danger. Important nerves passing through the muscles of the neck are protected while the nature of the threat is identified. When prolonged, it causes muscle tension and pain.*

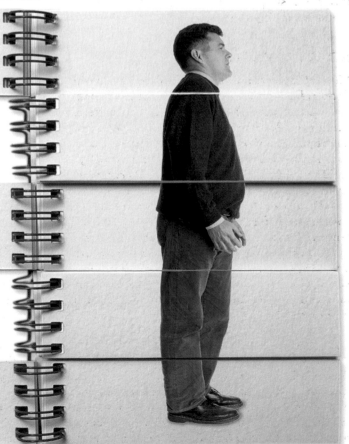

TILTING THE PELVIS *forward is an attempt to retreat as far as possible without moving the feet. It creates excessive low back tension and disturbs muscle antagonism so that the abdominal muscles lose tension and the vital organs tend to prolapse.*

LOCKING THE LEG MUSCLES *makes the knee joints less flexible, which prevents the body from collapsing and showing vulnerability. It often reveals the extreme effort involved in trying to cope with stress.*

FIT FOR MASSAGE: DIET

I N SPITE OF MANY claims to the contrary, massage is more successful when
used as a way of maintaining a healthy body than when used as a means
of combating the wear and tear created by unfitness. Lower back problems,
for example, can be greatly reduced by massage therapy if the patient can be
encouraged to lead a healthier life generally, but the most remedial forms of
massage have little lasting influence if the patient's body is basically unfit.
One of the main factors determining fitness is diet and the nutrition it provides.

NUTRITION IS A COMPLEX process to which massage
itself contributes at the microcosmic level. The
movements of massage improve the distribution of
the blood and help in the elimination of waste
products from the tissues. At the more familiar
macro level, the food we consume represents the raw
material of our diet, and the source of the nutrients
our bodies need for maintenance and activity.

In the developing world, people often struggle to
acquire enough food to nourish themselves, yet
where they can obtain enough food their diet is often
relatively good. The affluent societies, by contrast,
are embarrassed by a glut of food, yet paradoxically
this does not prevent malnutrition. Much of the food
we eat is denatured and refined, and in the process
valuable nutrients are lost. More significantly, the

NATURAL BODY EFFICIENCY

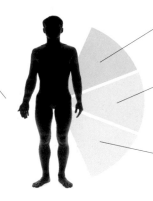

NATURAL WELL-BALANCED DIET
- **Energy:** *Total energy is provided
not only by selecting fresh food but
also by ensuring good respiration
and circulation.*
- **Healing Properties:** *It is almost
impossible to over-consume the natural
vitamins and minerals which initiate
healing responses.*
- **Weight Maintenance:** *Eating too
much fat, from any source, is the main
reason for becoming overweight.*

QUASI FOODS
*Foods which are claimed to possess
distinct nutritional properties, such
as "brain foods," are fraudulent.*

PROCESSED FOODS
*Convenience foods are convenient
only to manufacturers. They are
nutritionally inconvenient and
disadvantage the body.*

DIETING FOODS
*For foods to be truly diet foods they
should not be consumed at all.*

FLUID INTAKE

There is still much confusion over the value of fluids generally in
our diet. Some authorities recommend a high intake of water, but
others suggest that overconsumption disturbs the digestion of food and
is depleting because of the indigestion it causes. The high salt content
of the processed foods we eat also results in a tendency to retain fluid
in the body. Massage practitioners are aware of the consequences
of fluid retention, which include poor muscle tone and a
tendency to bruise easily. It is also a contributory factor in
raised blood pressure. The experience of athletes confirms that
a relatively low fluid intake can improve both strength and
stamina, suggesting that a moderate consumption of fluids is
the most healthy course.

poor balance of a diet based on such foods can result in a net loss of nutrition. Such malnourishment leads to poor development of the body and a poor response to treatment and healing.

Processed foods such as refined sugar slow up healing because some of the body's energy has to be redirected to deal with their intensity. The argument that they provide energy is spurious, because such energy is so short-lived: it lasts no longer than the burst of flame created by throwing sugar on a fire. By contrast, abstention from sugars, excepting the sugars contained in fruits, is known to accelerate healing by liberating the body's inherent energy.

Foods and drinks reputed to be stimulating can create the impression of helping the body, but this is because their potential toxicity challenges our nerves. Their effect may seem restorative, but this is not the same as the true restoration produced by fresh, unadulterated food.

Perhaps the most confusing aspect of our modern diet is the way in which "natural" foodstuffs are promoted as an answer to our health problems. Many of the ingredients of such foods are imported from far away, and have exotic-sounding names that suggest near-magical properties. In reality, though, acquiring foods to which we ordinarily do not have access simply shifts the emphasis away from freshness, which is one of the most important elements of a healthy diet. Similarly, the concept of "dieting" contradicts the body's natural appetite for good, honest foods. If your daily diet is balanced and healthy you will find no need for crash dieting.

FEAR AND ANXIETY

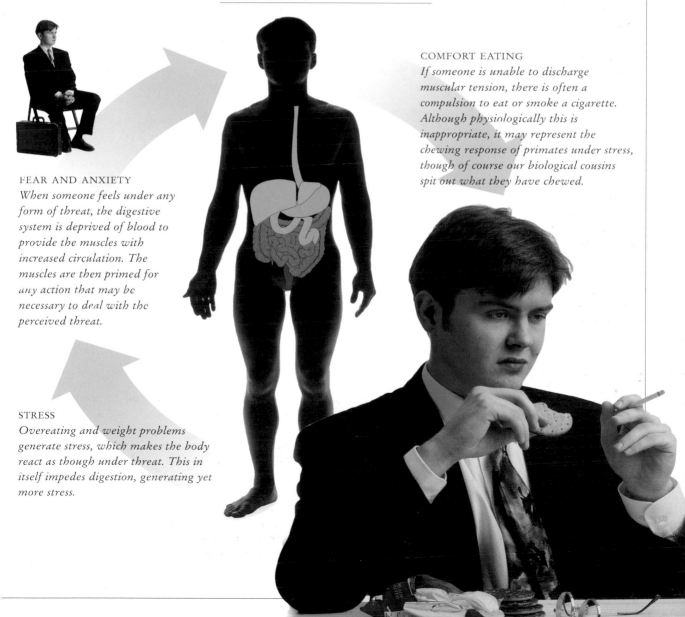

COMFORT EATING
If someone is unable to discharge muscular tension, there is often a compulsion to eat or smoke a cigarette. Although physiologically this is inappropriate, it may represent the chewing response of primates under stress, though of course our biological cousins spit out what they have chewed.

FEAR AND ANXIETY
When someone feels under any form of threat, the digestive system is deprived of blood to provide the muscles with increased circulation. The muscles are then primed for any action that may be necessary to deal with the perceived threat.

STRESS
Overeating and weight problems generate stress, which makes the body react as though under threat. This in itself impedes digestion, generating yet more stress.

THE SAFE TOUCH OF MASSAGE

THERE IS A DIRECT link between our enjoyment of physical contact and our deep memories of life in the womb, yet this reassuring association can be disrupted by later experiences. Inappropriate physical contact can be very confusing, since it may take the form of too much contact or too little. Those who have suffered its worst excesses sometimes feel disturbed by a sense of responsibility for the experience. It may be that, because touch is such an undeniable need, such people feel that they have been somehow misunderstood.

IF THE LEVEL OF received touch is insufficient, it brings little comfort and is so un-containing that it also brings no relief from tension. In such circumstances people often feel they have never enjoyed the strength of contact they need.

Little children are surprisingly trusting of contact with strangers. This might be because we are very dependent on physical contact for communication before our understanding of language develops. The need continues throughout life, for when people are lost for words, it seems natural to extend a reassuring hand as if to say "I understand you."

When we have no one available to provide this touch, we may seek the comfort of another physical sensation. For some people this leads to an abusive relationship with food. The act of eating when upset is unwise, since the digestive organs are unlikely to function properly under conditions of emotional disturbance. The resulting problems are familiar enough, but the underlying distress is easily obscured when the food consumption itself becomes an issue.

If someone has withdrawn from the world of physical contact because of unhappy experiences, the safe touch of massage may provide the solution. Any preconceptions that massage is actively given to a compliant, passive recipient are dispelled at the first treatment. Most people are pleasantly surprised at how involved they feel in their massage, while at the same time feeling increasingly at ease.

Massage treatment is gentle and yet provides a firm support. The practitioner has no expectations of the patient, but is guided by his or her responses. Their joint aim is to establish a trusting relationship, sharing a womb-like contact that has the potential to bring understanding and integration to the problems of the past.

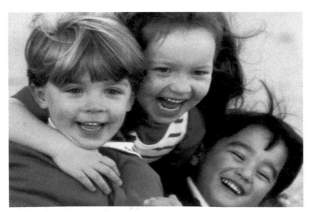

CHILDREN

Children normally enjoy massage. Young bodies have heightened sensitivity, and each stroke of massage offers an introduction to a variety of pressures, rhythms, and textures. The lighter effleurage strokes which stressed adults appreciate are often too tickly for tense children; they prefer soft, containing squeezes or slow stretches.

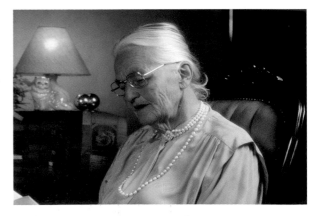

OLDER PEOPLE

Massage often induces reminiscence in older patients, and this means that massage can present a challenge to people who have survived a partner's death, since the caring touch of massage can magnify their loss. Yet many people have reported that massage is helpful with grieving, giving the support they needed to let their loved ones go.

AN INVITATION TO HEALTH

PEOPLE WHO ARE new to massage often express delight in their rediscovery of touch and movement – both as givers experiencing the heightened awareness of their sense of touch and creativity, and as receivers enjoying their capacity to respond. The benefits of this rediscovery are both physical and mental, emphasizing the way both aspects of health are interconnected. The theme of this book is an affirmation that our health is literally in our own hands, to be explored, relished, and enjoyed.

PHYSICALLY YOU HAVE to be reasonably fit to give a massage, but even those who have been suffering back problems are known to receive benefit from providing massage for others. This is because it increases postural awareness and develops economy of movement. Many muscles that are not normally used in everyday life are brought into play in giving massage. In particular, those of the legs and trunk become well-coordinated, and this helps people who spend much of their time sitting in office chairs.

Mentally, massagers learn how to relax as a treatment progresses, so that they find an almost meditative attitude emerging. This uncultivated state of mind creates an atmosphere that encourages the release of tension in the patient. Yet despite this relaxed atmosphere many people find massage positively energizing. The reason for this may lie in the release of nervous tension. The energy drain created by such tension can make you feel thoroughly depleted, both mentally and physically.

When the strokes of massage successfully deal with the tension, this locked up energy immediately becomes available. For some, this might manifest itself as a desire to tackle a long-overdue job, but paradoxically the release of energy can also lead to a long, deep, refreshing night's sleep.

Intellectually, reviewing the effects of massage satisfies our curiosity about how our bodies work helping to make some sense of our intricate physical, mental, and emotional lives. We are naturally inquisitive beings, able to take a detached view of our experience. Through massage we can understand how tension plays a significant part in health, and how hypertensions disturb the balance of our systems. The simple, gentle movements of massage demonstrate that cycles of tension can be interrupted, and positive rhythms of health reestablished.

HAND AND MIND

Massage is a supremely holistic therapy, in that it has both physical and mental benefits for giver and receiver. In the same way, learning the art of massage employs both the natural wisdom of the body and the received wisdom acquired by the intellect. The two are complementary, and while it is true that massage cannot be learned from books alone, it is equally true that hands-on experience by itself leads to an incomplete understanding of the way massage works and its potential for promoting health. One thing that massage teaches us is that body and mind are one, so do not fall into the trap of ignoring the intellect and assuming that your hands will teach you all you need to know. Your mind is an asset, like your hands. Use them both.

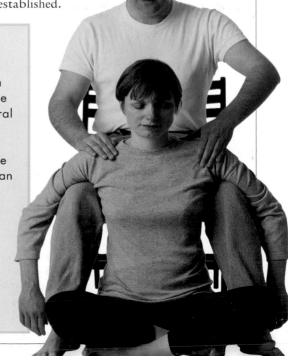

PROFESSIONAL TREATMENT

PROFESSIONAL MASSAGE IS not necessarily very different from the help you might get from an untrained enthusiast, except that it is formalized. The professional may not even be as experienced as a skilled amateur, but professional massage potentially offers more. This is because the way a massage practice is run intensifies the influence of treatment and can produce a very special relationship.

THE APPOINTMENT

Anyone requiring professional help of any kind usually starts by making an appointment to be seen. Appointments, of course, provide a practical way for the therapist to manage the practice, but for the patient the arrangement immediately begins to have a positive effect. Simply securing an appointment is in itself very reassuring. The appointment also offers an opportunity to be heard and examined, and to have one's problem generally witnessed. The appointment defines the length of time with the therapist, which gives the patient the reassurance of feeling contained, no matter how serious the problem might be.

THE TREATMENT ROOM

The atmosphere created by the decor of the treatment room makes an important contribution to the effectiveness of the treatment itself. It is a strong statement, a reflection of the practitioner and his or her philosophy. The room may appear to be a clinical space, where analytic experiences occur; it may look like a studio, designed for creative expression; it may have the trappings of a temple for revelations; it may be a comfortable-looking place designed to make the patient feel safe.

The appearance of the practitioner may reflect the decor of the room, but not always. Occasionally, practitioners have trouble reconciling their own taste with the image they want to project, exemplified by the dilemma over what to wear. White coats are relics of early surgical practice where protective clothing was essential. Modern, clinical tunics are neater and high-buttoned, a point that has not been lost on observers of the consultation process. The patient may be nearly naked, but the practitioner is clothed right up to the chin. Apparently, patients do prefer their practitioners to wear predictable clothing, but not necessarily formal clinical attire. It is enough that the practitioner appears in similar clothes from consultation to consultation. Many patients are unnerved by radical changes in appearance, and respond in the same way if the furnishings are moved around or replaced. Some practitioners feel that it is important to dress similarly to their patients, with perhaps simply a small professional lapel badge to signify that they are at work.

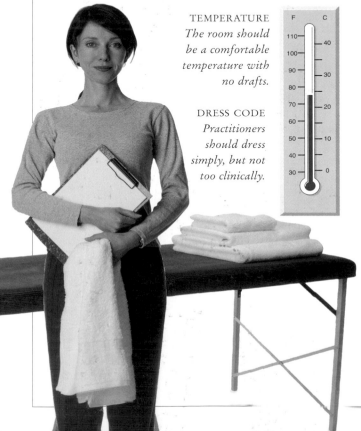

TEMPERATURE
The room should be a comfortable temperature with no drafts.

DRESS CODE
Practitioners should dress simply, but not too clinically.

DECOR AND EQUIPMENT
The equipment should be clean and efficient, but beyond this, the decor of *the consulting room will be a reflection of the practitioner's personal style and philosophy.*

MASSAGE THERAPISTS DO NOT...

- diagnose medical conditions unless medically qualified
- give treatment or advice for conditions in which they do not hold appropriate qualifications
- prescribe drugs or pharmaceutically active products
- criticize fellow practitioners
- practice without adequate insurance cover
- behave in any way that would bring grief upon themselves or bring the profession into disrepute
- continue in massage practice if guilty of a breach of the Code of Conduct

MASSAGE THERAPISTS DO...

- assess medical conditions for suitability of massage treatment
- refer to qualified practitioners' conditions for which massage is contraindicated
- gain qualifications to dispense and massage with aromatic plant oils
- act honorably toward patients, colleagues, and other health professionals
- hold insurance cover that offers professional and public liability
- conduct their professional lives with propriety and dignity at all times
- maintain standards of conduct within their practice that are beyond reproach

Any changes in the atmosphere of the treatment room or disruption of treatment routine can be upsetting to the progress of a patient, whether or not this is consciously acknowledged.

THE FIRST CONSULTATION

Patients who have already been through orthodox consultation usually have a lengthy case history. It may seem tiresome or intrusive to have to divulge much of this information to the practitioner. However, whereas conventional methods aim at securing a diagnosis, a massage practitioner is concerned with understanding the story implied by the case history. Only by appreciating the problem from the patient's and, more often, the patient's body's point of view, can the practitioner decide on an appropriate massage treatment.

The patient may well be nervous at first meeting the practitioner, and naturally apprehensive about removing clothing. Sensitive practitioners do not make assumptions that people are experienced patients just because they have consulted several times or have a long-standing problem. In the same way that a request for information is put in terms of "I need to know if you are on any medication," so a request to undress might begin "In order to treat your shoulder I need you to take off your shirt."

It is important to give accurate information. The practitioner relies on the information given at this and subsequent consultations to assess whether there are any reasons to modify the treatment. It is very rare that massage is completely unsuitable for medical reasons, but the practitioner may feel that

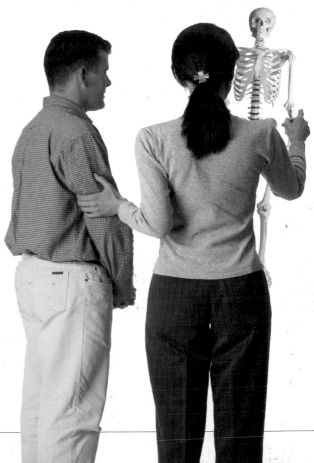

FIRST CONSULTATION
The first encounter is largely devoted to a process of mutual discovery. While the practitioner identifies the problems that have prompted the consultation the patient has a chance to assess the practitioner.

applying massage while the patient is undergoing another type of treatment is undesirable, and in this case the appointment may be postponed.

POST-CONSULTATION

Both therapist and patient need time to appreciate the impact of the first consultation, and the therapist will suggest a suitable interlude before the next meeting. For practical reasons the patient might like to be offered a plan of treatment, but although the practitioner may believe that the problem can be dealt with in a precise number of sessions, he or she may prefer not to communicate this to the patient.

The main thing to decide is whether there is any advantage in continuing the treatment. This is both a professional and personal decision for, in common with other complementary therapies, massage deals in relationships as well as clinical technicalities.

When patients are asked, by friends, whether massage treatment has cured a problem, they often describe feeling better, easier, or more positive, rather than less painful or more flexible. This emotional, rather than analytical response reflects the importance of the understanding between patient and therapist, and indicates the patient's underlying confidence in the process of relating. On the practitioner's part, there is obviously great satisfaction to be gained from seeing quick results, but most massage therapists take a long, almost evolutionary view of progress, and enjoy the process of caring as much as the achievement of curing.

PROFESSIONAL MISCONDUCT

Failure to observe professional guidelines – by practitioner or client – is demeaning and compromising for both. It is just as unacceptable for the patient to try to extract extra time if treatments feel beneficial as for the practitioner to offer free treatments to enjoy their company. A practitioner and patient may already be friends, or become friends, but within the treatment session they must aim to relate in an organized way, rather like the players in a team. Otherwise, the treatment is in danger of losing its specialness. Professionalism does not make massage practice impersonal or distant; on the contrary, it defines and preserves the usefulness of the relationship.

Practitioners, as custodians of the professional relationship, aim to educate their patients' sometimes unintentional misconduct. They can also discuss unexpected or troubling responses with their colleagues. Patients, on the other hand, enter the consultation in deep trust and are less likely, for a variety of reasons, to perceive unprofessional behavior in the practitioner. Furthermore, patients may not have the opportunity to discuss any such problems with family or friends because they have sought treatment confidentially. For these reasons, and in the interest of other patients, any misconduct should always be reported to regulatory bodies.

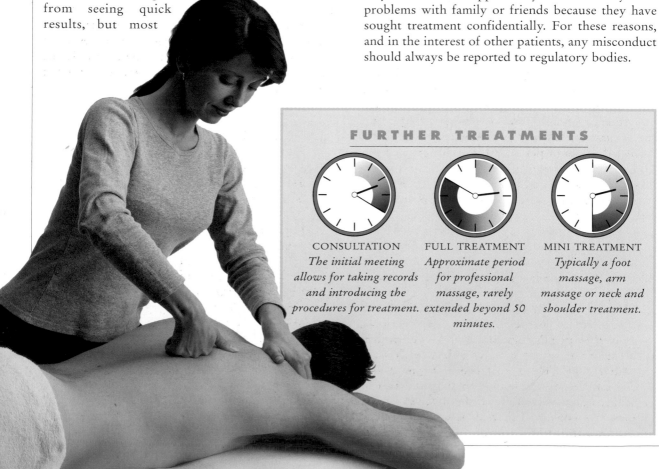

FURTHER TREATMENTS

CONSULTATION
The initial meeting allows for taking records and introducing the procedures for treatment.

FULL TREATMENT
Approximate period for professional massage, rarely extended beyond 50 minutes.

MINI TREATMENT
Typically a foot massage, arm massage or neck and shoulder treatment.

FINDING A PRACTITIONER

OBTAINING PROFESSIONAL massage is quite different from seeking conventional healthcare. Complementary practice may be scarce in your area, or you may hear of practitioners only to discover that they are not professionally organized. Furthermore, the reasons for choosing complementary therapy are usually much more personal than having conventional treatment, and consequently the personality of the practitioner will be significant.

WHEN YOU FIND a practitioner, you will want to check his or her professional credentials. It is very likely that an advertising practitioner will have a certain level of training in massage therapy. This may have been acquired as part of a wider discipline such as yoga; it may have been obtained on an extended, physiologically based course; or it may have been the subject of a postgraduate medical course. All of these can provide good training, but it is not always easy to check the standard achieved because standards in professional massage are not unified, either internationally or within many countries. One set of standards that can be trusted is that of the International Therapy Examination Council (ITEC), which is based in Great Britain; these standards are recognized worldwide as qualifications for complementary therapists.

Another concern for the patient is the therapist's degree and quality of experience. A qualification may be reassuring, but when was it obtained? In this connection, more does not necessarily mean better, for although practice perfects technique, keeping up with new trends and developments, updating knowledge and periodically refreshing basic concepts are important disciplines in health work. Regularly updated techniques can be a far better measure of a practitioner's professional commitment than a list of academic qualifications.

SAFEGUARDS

Before a therapist can charge fees, he or she must be properly insured. The insurance cover is usually obtained by therapists on qualification, and it offers protection to both parties.

From the patient's point of view, however, the real insurance is the fact that the practitioner belongs to a regulating body. These professional organizations are, of course, set up mainly for the protection of their members. Their ethical codes precisely define professional aims and behavior, however, and these ultimately safeguard the patient.

A massage practitioner may choose not to belong to an existing professional body, either for philosophical reasons or because there is local disunity. If so, be sure you are satisfied with the explanation before proceeding to treatment. You could ask for a practitioner's "Code of Ethics" to be sent to you before making your initial appointment.

MAKING A CHOICE

Complementary therapy is as much about who performs the treatment as the actual nature of the treatment itself. This explains why a sensitive, newly qualified massage practitioner can be just as effective as an experienced colleague, even in complex cases.

It is the relationship between the participants that permits the benefits of massage to be experienced and for this reason, all other considerations aside, the most reliable guide to finding a practitioner is the personal recommendation of others.

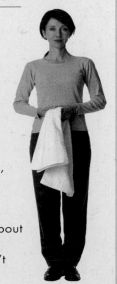

CHECKLIST

- Ask friends, doctors, and hospitals for recommended practitioners.
- Go to the public library for a Register of Massage Practitioners.
- Ask a massage practice for a copy of their Code of Ethics before making an appointment. If unavailable, speak to the practitioner personally.
- As your first treatment approaches, don't worry about trying to be relaxed with someone you trust, but don't know. You will be.

THE CASE RECORD

Massage therapy is increasingly finding a place in general healthcare through the agency of conventional treatments such as midwifery and hospice care, but many people experience massage therapy for the first time at the hands of a practitioner, after consulting in his or her own right.

A MAJOR REASON why people seek such therapy is because they perceive it to be truly complementary to the best of other healthcare options. This means that if you make a private appointment yourself, you will almost certainly have experience of conventional therapies. If this is your first experience of complementary medicine, you may have to adapt to a wider, more democratic treatment style than the one you have been used to.

All massage therapists are likely to take an approach that suits their individual style, rather than follow a prescribed method like a conventional practitioner. In common with their orthodox colleagues, however, they may invite you to help complete a formal case record document. You might be irritated if you have already documented your details many times before, especially if you have found the experience more alienating than useful.

A complementary case record is not compiled for the exclusive benefit of the practitioner. It is information to be shared between you, for your joint consideration and reflection: an illustrated version is given here.

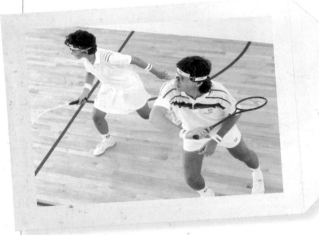

RECREATION
Finding out how you offset the effects of your occupation and life's routine will be useful to the practitioner.

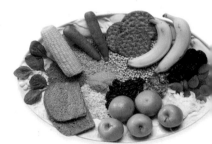

DIET
This is not itemized, but your attitudes to food may reflect how you look after yourself.

PROFESSION
The practitioner will want to assess whether your occupation is subjecting you to repetitive strain.

MEASUREMENTS

Either you or the practitioner may choose to have your physical statistics recorded at the first consultation. Many therapists feel that taking such clinical measurements reinforces the impression made by a patient. On your own part, you may like to use the readings as a baseline for measuring the benefits of treatment. One problem with any measurement, though, is that it can be used as a basis of comparison with an unattainable ideal, rather than a measure of personal wellbeing.

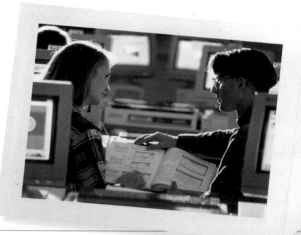

STRICTLY CONFIDENTIAL

PRESENTING SYMPTOMS

This gives the reason for the appointment. It is literally what you "present" the practitioner, as if to say "take this from me." This can be recorded as a list of symptoms in your own words, such as "bad headaches and flashing lights." Alternatively a diagnosed condition may be set down in inverted commas, such as "migraine."

MEDICAL HISTORY AND MEDICINES: SURGERY: GENERAL PRACTITIONER

It is very important that you give information on any current treatments you may be having (especially long-term medication) or any recent operations (if you have been anesthetized) before having massage treatment. It helps your practitioner decide your suitability for massage. With your permission, it may be necessary to consult with your doctor before massage is given.

MEDICAL CONDITIONS

Perhaps you suffer from a sub-clinical condition such as rheumatism which, although not attracting medical intervention, nonetheless reduces your quality of life. Such conditions are often easier to describe in terms of the system which they affect, as follows:

DIGESTIVE, CIRCULATORY, NERVOUS, MUSCLES/BONES, MENSTRUAL CYCLE

HEIGHT, WEIGHT, BLOOD PRESSURE

These are basic elements of any health check, since they are valuable indicators of life-threatening conditions.

JOINT FLEXIBILITY

These freely-movable joints are tested for flexibility as an indicator of the general state of tension in your body.

SPINAL POSTURE: FORWARD, BACKWARD, LEFT TURN, RIGHT TURN, SIDEWAYS LEFT/RIGHT

Your spinal posture is observed for general fitness and possible pressure on nerves.

SKIN SEGMENTATION BOX

This is a diagrammatic aid for swiftly recording any areas of pain or discomfort.

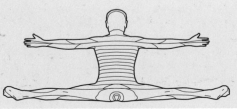

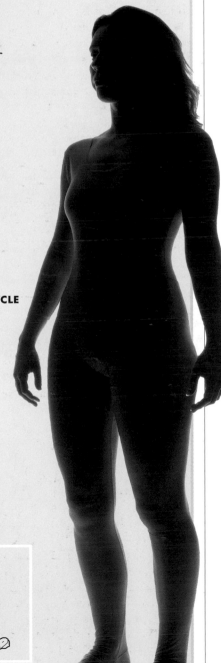

MASSAGE AT HOME

THERE IS AN ATTITUDE, even among complementary health schools, that only trained professionals are competent to treat others. This goes against the tradition of natural therapy, much of which is derived from enlightened home care. In many cultures, the grandparents were the custodians of family healthcare, and this wisdom was passed down through the generations. The intention of this book is to build on this tradition and emphasize the humanistic as well as the technical aspects of massage. It aims to encourage a communicative experience, rather like teaching a friend to swim.

THERE ARE MANY opportunities to use massage in the home – with fractious children, for stressed and exhausted parents, and with infirm or incapacitated older relatives.

Home massage has the advantage of being available without delay. Brief treatments can be given more frequently, which increases the benefits of the simplest form of massage. It is also possible to combine massage with bathing, which is very refreshing, and enjoy immediate rest after a treatment session.

Massage can increase reassuring contact when children are frightened by respiratory illnesses such as asthma. Potentially chronic conditions, such as the lower back pain that may develop from pregnancy, can be treated daily. If someone is immobilized by an accident or injury, simple foot or neck massage can help the patient keep a clear head.

Sometimes massage in families doesn't work. There can be a conflict between the intimacy that normally exists between family members and the sense of detachment that massaging brings. What begins as a relaxed, supportive session can become uncomfortable as your intimate feels an unusual distance developing.

Friends and family can also find it difficult to take up a half-hearted offer of massage if the massager is still building confidence. So be positive in your approach and confident of your skill. If you have any doubts about suitability for massage, refer to a qualified practitioner, who should be only too willing to encourage your efforts.

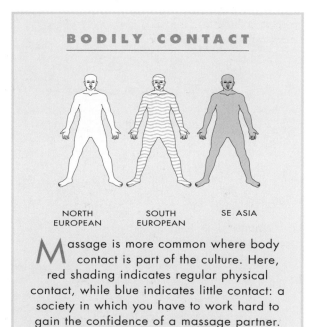

BODILY CONTACT

NORTH EUROPEAN   SOUTH EUROPEAN   SE ASIA

Massage is more common where body contact is part of the culture. Here, red shading indicates regular physical contact, while blue indicates little contact: a society in which you have to work hard to gain the confidence of a massage partner.

MASSAGE AT HOME
Although the setting may seem less than ideal, massage at home offers many benefits. One of the most valuable of these is immediacy: people with chronic problems can be treated daily, if needed.

ENCOUNTER OR CONFRONTATION?

IN MANY CULTURES, adults tend to associate the intimacy of touch with the intimacy of sex. This creates the dilemma, both for receivers and givers of massage, of reconciling sexuality with the physicality of massage. This is not a unique problem, since research suggests that the subject of sex occupies much adult thinking time. Sexual issues can arise in all human encounters, and are almost bound to arise during a massage session.

JUST AS IN OTHER situations, the process of clearing away any sexual ambiguity in massage starts with an awareness of your own individual sexual consciousness. If this consciousness has been repressed, you can be sure that it will awaken as your interest in massage grows. This can come as a shock to promising massagers, and even if you consider that your attitude toward sex is liberal, you will find that it is soon put to the test.

It is not always possible to know when a personal encounter is becoming sexualized. Many sexual responses take place at subconscious levels, and while your massages are intended to be

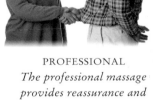

pleasurable experiences, you may never know the quality of the sensation your partner is experiencing.

Don't worry. Massage offers an opportunity of honestly addressing sexuality, and your partner's embarrassment or naivety may be only mirroring your own. The sensual element forms the basis of the unspoken rapport in massage, and for experienced practitioners sensuality is an important aspect of the therapeutic relationship. The more experience you gain in massage the more reassuring your touch will become. Your partner will respond accordingly, and the sexuality dilemma will evaporate.

PROFESSIONAL
The professional massage provides reassurance and confirms needs.

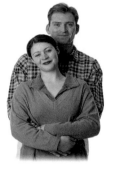

LOVERS
Lovers specialize in unstructured, spontaneous massage.

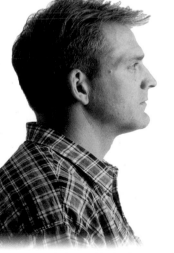

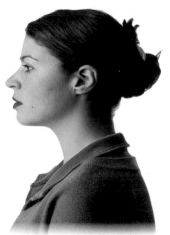

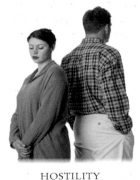

HOSTILITY
Avoid misunderstandings by clarifying what you expect from massage.

ENCOUNTER
For many people, massage offers the opportunity for genuine human contact. It does not matter that their partner may be a complete stranger, since the contact has the potential to be fleeting, intense, and unconditional.

CONFRONTATION
For some, massage will represent a challenging experience as the submission of control and extension of trust involved is considerable. For the giver, the prospect of being responsible for another's wellbeing can be quite daunting.

CASE STUDY 3

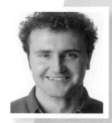

Name: Paul
Age: 32
Personal circumstances: Married; 1 child
Medical history: No problems
Presenting: Stress
Referred by: Self

NOTES

- Paul is the elder of two brothers.
- He manages a small electronics firm and aims to keep fit by running along the nearby beach as often as possible.
- He takes the responsibilities of his job very seriously and finds it increasingly difficult to forget them at home.
- His father suffered from high blood pressure before dying in his fifties.

PAUL'S ATTENTION was drawn to massage by an article in a men's health magazine. He wasn't sure at this stage if he was suited to massage, but despite this he somewhat hesitantly joined an introductory 10-week massage course at a local center, hoping that this would provide him with regular massage that might help with the stress of work. In the event, he was to discover that the act of giving massage would prove more therapeutic than receiving it.

ANY APPREHENSION Paul had about his course was dispelled when he met the other participants, many of whom were in a similarly stressed condition. Paul enjoyed the part of the course that explained about the effects of stress on the body, and he was soon able to appreciate why he had been feeling so irritable.

He was surprised to find that his initial response to being massaged was to fall asleep. Although this was a relaxing experience, he felt that he was missing out: he wanted to learn about what was happening to him during massage, rather than drift into sleep. The instructor reassured him that the sleep reaction was not unusual in a stressed person.

It took some weeks for Paul to notice that he felt as good, if not better, after giving someone else a massage. The instructor had explained the beneficial effect of massage on the giver, but Paul had been too preoccupied with his reaction to being massaged to hear it. Gradually, however, he realized that he was looking forward to giving massages. Rather than seeking the relaxed nervous oblivion he had initially craved, he discovered that that he was enjoying the focus of concentration necessary to give effective massage.

Physically, Paul felt energetic, more at ease, and fresher through giving massage. He had fewer problems with headaches and backaches, and slept better.

He was able to practice massage with his family, who found that since attending the massage course Paul was able to give more of himself at home.

At work he felt less pressure to take control, especially where this involved human relations. He was more flexible in his attitudes and less aggressive in his approach to daily problems.

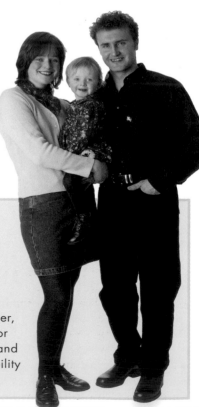

HOW DID MASSAGE HELP?

People such as Paul, who are being overrun by their sense of responsibility, find it hard to release themselves to the relaxing effects of massage treatment, and it is significant that Paul decided to attend a massage class rather than make an appointment with a practitioner. This enabled him to discover his own ability as a massager, and the benefits of giving massage. He developed an attentive care for others that countered the carelessness that was emerging in his work and family relationships. He was able to adjust his tension by using his ability as a manager to "manage" the tensions in those he massaged.

CASE STUDY 4

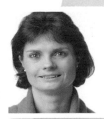

JAN LEARNED from a midwife colleague that a massage support group was being organized for hospital staff. She recalled that during her training she had worked alongside physiotherapists in the obstetric department of the hospital, but had never been particularly drawn to rehabilitation medicine. However, the idea of supporting a new staff group attracted her and she decided to attend.

Name: Jan
Age: 23
Personal circumstances: Single
Medical history: No problems
Presenting: Fatigue
Referred by: Self

NOTES
• Jan is a nurse on a busy ward in a large teaching hospital.
• She finds her job challenging but she is dedicated to her career in caring and goes to work energetically.
• She has begun to feel very tired by the end of her shift and has noticed that she occasionally feels depressed for no obvious reason.

SYMPTOMS	ASSESSMENT	TREATMENT
• Tiredness • Depression	• Overwork • Difficulty in letting go and expressing her emotions.	• Simply experiencing the touch of massage provided Jan with an insight into her own problems, as well as a new interest.

AT THE FIRST meeting Jan was interested to hear the teacher emphasize the importance of the quality of touch in massage. Although clearly having aspects in common with the physiotherapy she had previously witnessed, massage was being presented as something to do with communication. She began to wonder if massage might not be a good idea for the patients in the hospital ward.

The second session introduced massage of the neck and shoulders. Colleagues partnered off and Jan eagerly opted to give massage first. She followed the instructions diligently, but toward the end of the sequence she noticed that she was tiring, and was relieved to exchange places and sit down to be massaged.

As her massage began, she suddenly felt very exhausted, and was shocked to find that tears were welling up inside her. She didn't have the energy to pull herself together and somehow she didn't care. She was aware of the massage teacher by her side, encouraging her partner to massage her with slow, warm stroking. After what seemed like a short time in this unfamiliar emotional state, Jan noticed she was starting to breathe deeply. She felt a little shaky at the end of her massage, but she thanked her partner. She returned home and was relieved to go straight to bed.

Yet in the morning she awoke feeling better than she could ever remember.

CARE FOR THE CARER
Looking after other people is stressful in itself, and even carers need to be cared for.

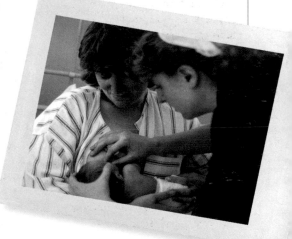

HOW DID MASSAGE HELP?

Jan's experience of massage made her aware of the need to relax her self-control and feel the caring attention that she so generously gave to others. She never cried again at the sessions, but did so at other times – something that had formerly been a rare event. She enjoyed giving her colleagues massage, but knew that the benefits of being massaged perfectly complemented her work as a carer. She abandoned her plan to provide massage for her patients, and instead became an enthusiastic promoter of the staff support group.

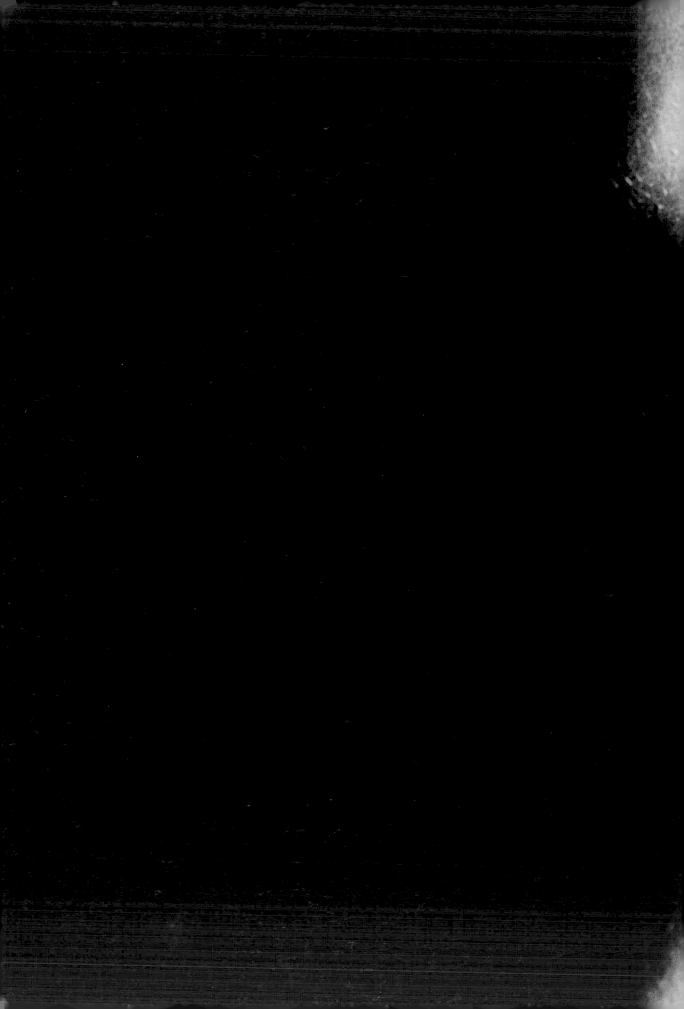

PART TWO

Understanding your Body

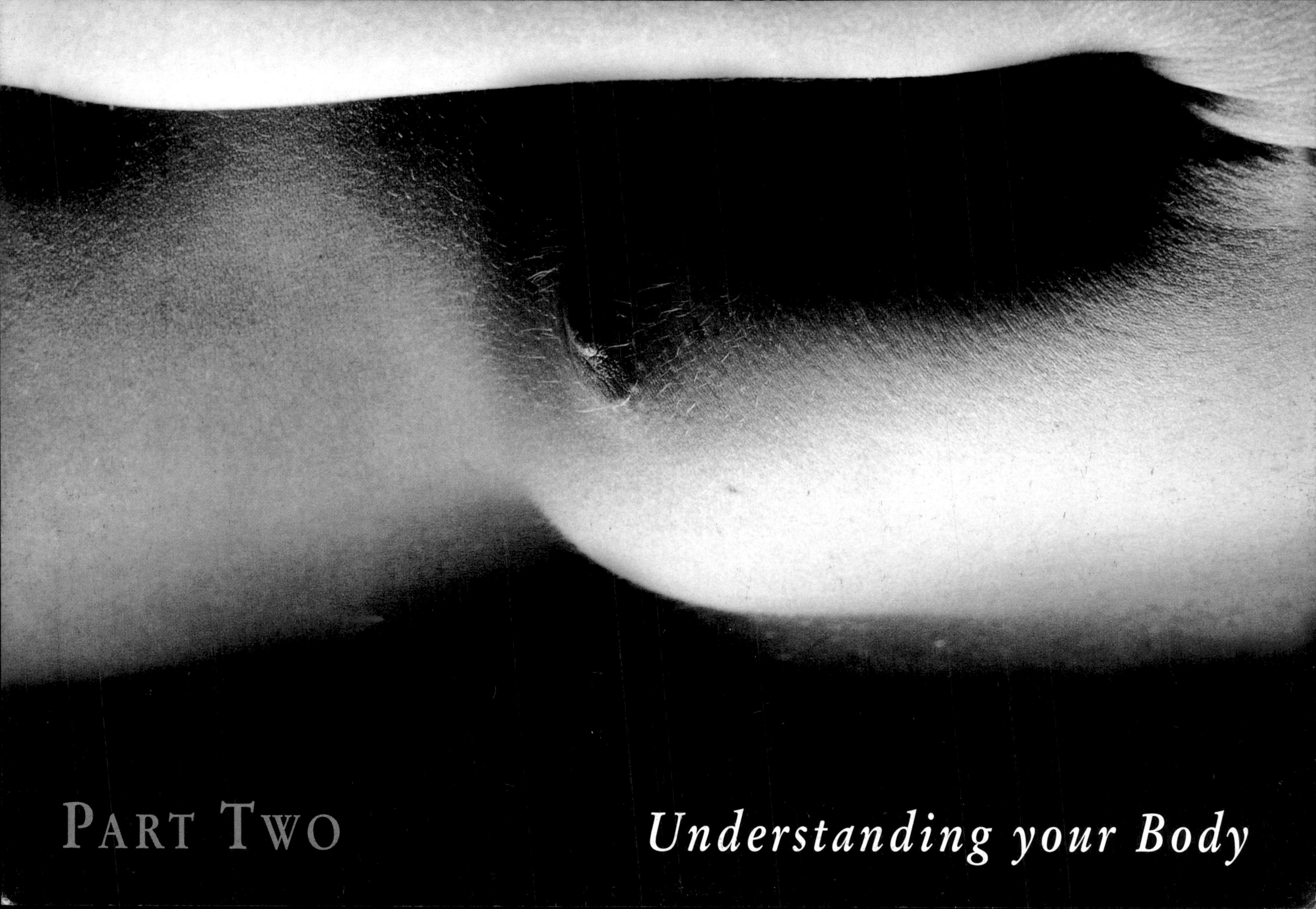

ANATOMY OF MOVEMENT

A GOOD GRASP OF basic anatomy is essential to massage. Understanding the body's basic structures will contribute to your sensitivity toward it, and help you deal with the deeper, more persistent tensions suffered by your massage partners. By learning how the body works, you will dispel some of the myths created by experts whose terminology has tended to make the whole subject their exclusive domain. Your body is your concern; it is up to you to find out about it.

MANY MASSAGERS RESIST the study of anatomy, because they see it as part of conventional medical practice, and somehow inappropriate to a holistic therapy like massage. It can also be frustrating trying to integrate an intellectual understanding of the body with more intuitive feelings for massage. This resistance is worth trying to overcome, since the more you massage, the more you will want to know what is happening to the body you are massaging.

The body is an extremely complex organism, and acquiring a full understanding of its mechanisms can take several years. Luckily, a full understanding is not necessary for massage. You can learn a great deal about the body from observing everyday movements. Notice the different ways people get in and out of cars or catch falling objects: knowledge gained in this way is just as relevant to massage as reading about muscle action in books.

The theory has its place, though, and on the ensuing pages the way the bones, joints, and muscles interact in the body is described in some detail. The essential thing is to grasp the way all this fits and works together, to create a vivid picture of the moving body beneath the skin.

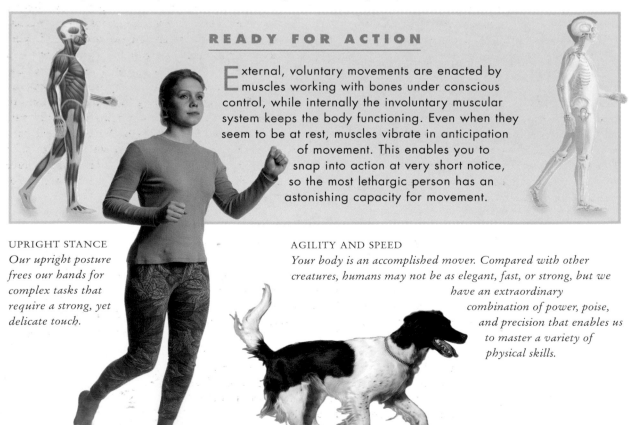

READY FOR ACTION

External, voluntary movements are enacted by muscles working with bones under conscious control, while internally the involuntary muscular system keeps the body functioning. Even when they seem to be at rest, muscles vibrate in anticipation of movement. This enables you to snap into action at very short notice, so the most lethargic person has an astonishing capacity for movement.

UPRIGHT STANCE
Our upright posture frees our hands for complex tasks that require a strong, yet delicate touch.

AGILITY AND SPEED
Your body is an accomplished mover. Compared with other creatures, humans may not be as elegant, fast, or strong, but we have an extraordinary combination of power, poise, and precision that enables us to master a variety of physical skills.

THE HUMAN FRAME

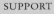

Architecturally, the human frame is a walking tower of three stories. The top story is the skull, which contains the brain and most of the sense organs. The middle story is the chest, which houses the heart and respiratory organs. The lower story is the abdomen, which contains the digestive apparatus. The proportions of the body are as precise as an architect's drawing. If the arms are extended, their span corresponds to the height of the body. The spine is three times the height of the head, the arm is three times the length of the hand, and the leg is three times the length of the foot. The ancient Egyptians recorded the height of the whole body as 19 times the length of the middle finger. We all recognize the beauty of those in whom these proportions are purely embodied.

SUPPORT
The skeleton is the internal scaffolding of the body. Without it, the body would be unable to support its weight or maintain its shape.

PROTECTION
Individual bones act like armor for the vital parts of the body. The brain, for example, is encased in a shell-like skull, and the heart and lungs are protected by a flexible cage of bones called the thorax.

LOCOMOTION
The numerous bones of the skeleton are articulated by a variety of joints that enable it to accomplish an immense variety of physical tasks.

THE SPINE

The spine is composed of 33 ring-like bones called vertebrae, which are stacked one upon the other to form the vertebral column. The cervical or neck vertebrae carry the weight of the head, while the more robust thoracic or chest vertebrae support the chest. The big lumbar vertebrae at the waist support the abdomen.

The elegant curves of the column are created by sitting, crawling, and learning to walk in childhood, and they are essential to our upright posture. The curvature absorbs all the shock to the skeleton caused by walking on two legs, especially over unyielding urban surfaces, and low back pain is more likely to be caused by loss of this curvature than by any intrinsic drawback of our upright stance.

Back pain is also associated with excessive curvature, known as spinal deviation, which is often brought about by occupational or recreational strain. The spine may also be disordered owing to a congenital defect. Typically, the lumbar spine carries over hyperextension from childhood, producing a problem known as lordosis. As people get older the thoracic spine has a tendency to kyphosis, or stiffening and hunching forwards. And even in the prime of life, normal right-side or left-side preference with the hand or foot can lead to a lateral deviation of the spine known as scoliosis. In all cases, massage with mobilization helps reduce spinal deviation and can alleviate the discomfort of well-established conditions.

THE FLEXIBLE SPINE

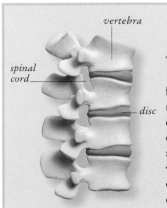

vertebra

spinal cord

disc

The joints between each bone in the spine permit only a small amount of movement, yet because they are multifaceted there are 150 articulations available. This makes the spine extremely flexible. Gymnasts who appear to be "double-jointed" are actually displaying normal flexibility. The neck vertebrae should be able to move particularly freely; without moving your shoulders, you should be able to swivel your head far enough in each direction to see all around you.

Legs and Pelvis

THE PELVIS IS a basin-like structure formed from two symmetrically encircling groups of bones that fuse together after birth. Its main role is to articulate the thigh bones and provide an anchor for the muscles of the spine and legs, so it is fundamental to locomotion in an upright posture. The pelvis is popularly associated with birth, since the female pelvis is thought to be wider than the male's to accommodate childbearing. In reality, though, it is the depth, front to back, of the pelvis that is of vital importance, and the body can make adjustments to this while the birth is actually in progress.

WE TEND TO REGARD the pelvis as an arrangement of sitting bones perfectly adapted for sitting on chairs, but in many cultures – and in infancy – people follow their natural instinct to squat rather than sit. This instinct is well-founded, for misusing the pelvis as a seat involves pressure on the wedge of spine within it – the coccyx – and disturbance to the spinal curves above. It may not be coincidental that problems of back disorder, menstrual and other abdominal complaints, as well as prematurely degenerative conditions of the legs, are less common within cultures that continue squatting in adult life. There have been many innovative attempts to create a more pelvic-friendly chair for the Western way of sitting, but without much success, for the perfect chair would have no seat.

PELVIC POSTURE

Placing more of the body's weight on one foot is confirmation of a pelvic problem. The pelvis rotates forward, and the body accommodates this with a forward rotation of the opposite shoulder to keep the head and neck in alignment with the base of the spine.

PELVIS
A rotated pelvis draws the spine into a spiral. This is felt as "hollow back."

KNEE
The knee is flexed on the affected side.

LEGS
Single leg bends are often much in evidence on the beach or around pools, confirming the widespread incidence of postural discomfort.

LEG-CROSSING

The body will accept the conventional seating arrangement for short periods, but eventually it starts to protest. It is fascinating that the common response to this discomfort is to adopt an even more bizarre posture. Leg-crossing could hardly be bettered as a way of magnifying the distress caused by overstaying the welcome of a chair. When loss of sensation ultimately produces deeper pain, many people just cross their legs the other way. When this too begins to cause pain, the sufferer typically struggles to stand up, while complaining about his or her legs.

The obvious pain that the legs suffer from leg-crossing is merely an urgent, conscious indication of far-reaching strains occurring throughout the body. Crossing the legs tilts and twists the pelvis, completing the partial collapse of abdominal posture caused by the body's contact with the back of the chair. Internally, the breathing is depressed and the abdomen becomes congested. The drag on the tail of the spine has to be compensated for by increased neck tension so that the head remains in a balanced position. Try to avoid it.

Head and Neck

IT IS A CURIOUS fact that a mouse, a giraffe, and a human all share the evolutionary distinction of having seven neck vertebrae. The way that the head is balanced on those vertebrae, however, is unique to the human body, and permits an unusual degree of mobility. To maintain this head posture, complex groups of muscles in the neck have to be held in tension all through a person's waking hours. At the same time, the subtler muscles of the neck are free to perform the graceful bending and rotational movements which contribute to gesture and self-expression.

THE SUCCESSFUL mechanical organization of the neck is vital in other ways, since it allows unimpeded functioning of the crucial nerves and blood vessels that pass between the brain and the rest of the body, as well as the digestive tract and airway.

Given this physiology, it might be expected that conventional healthcare would have recognized the importance of the neck to disorders of the body in general. This has not been so, and our understanding of the role of the neck

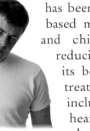

Tension in the neck is recognized as a factor in many disorders.

has been largely developed by manipulation-based massage therapies such as osteopathy and chiropractic. Therapies that involve reducing tension in the neck and realigning its bony relationships have been used to treat a wide variety of functional disorders including indigestion, palpitations of the heart, and laryngitis. Local pressures in the neck can lead to local problems such as headaches, or distant complaints such as numbness in the extremities, and these also respond to manipulative massage.

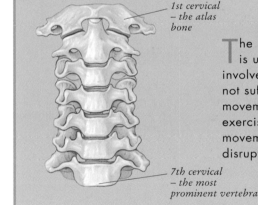

1st cervical – the atlas bone

7th cervical – the most prominent vertebra

THE BONES OF THE NECK

The seven bones of the neck allow considerable flexibility, but it is unwise to encourage this by neck-rolling exercises that involve deep backward bending. There are few people who have not suffered mild whiplash-type injury to the neck, and encircling movements can irritate the traumatized mid-joints. Also, unless the exercises are slow and deliberate repetitions of normal movements, there is a danger of fainting through disruption of the blood supply to the brain.

NERVOUS CONTROL

Most of the nerve tissue passing through the neck is safely enclosed by the vertebrae as the spinal cord, but 12 pairs of nerves issuing directly from the brain are routed through neck muscle. Most of these – the cranial nerves – lead to the head and face, but the tenth nerve – the vagus nerve – wanders down through the neck to the chest and abdomen.

The vagus exerts a calming influence on the body, and simple massage near the side of the neck encourages its action. Yet it can be overdone, so it is sometimes better to stimulate the vagus indirectly by massaging the nerve endings of the cranials in the head and face; this reflexes gently back to the vagus.

THE VAGUS NERVE
Gentle massage of the sides of the neck stimulates the vagus nerve and has a calming effect.

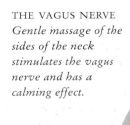

THE SKELETON

LOOK CLOSELY AT the skeleton, and it becomes apparent that human beings are not what they seem to be. The skull is so large, its eye sockets so deep. The pelvis has a depth and roundness that comes as something of a surprise. Comparing the living and skeletal hand is puzzling until you realize that the knuckles of each hand are the terminations of the palm bones. These confusions arise because we deduce the shapes of bones in the living body from prominent points like the hips, and these anatomical landmarks give little insight into the proportions of the skeleton itself.

THE LITERAL TRANSLATION of the word skeleton as "dried up" is misleading when applied to living bones. A typical long bone such as the femur is full of blood, and the bone marrow at its core produces the very cells of which all blood is composed. The marrow is surrounded by lightweight spongy bone and this in turn is enclosed by the dense material that forms the bone's compact exterior, rather like bamboo cane. This essentially tubular construction is extremely strong for its weight, and its ability to withstand stress compares favorably with the capacity of oak wood.

Bone is an evolving tissue that begins life as flexible cartilage, and with the arrival of blood and nutrients develops its characteristic boniness – a process known as ossification. As it matures, bone also grows. An adult is over three times the height of a newborn child, and all this growth has to be accommodated by extension of the bones. This is achieved by special cartilage cells that add material to the ends of the long bones and are gradually ossified in their turn. The bone depends on an adequate supply of calcium for this ossification process, and forms a convenient store of calcium for other body requirements.

At the age of about 20 the skeleton stops growing, and most of the cartilage in the growth zones becomes ossified. The skeleton does not ossify completely, though. Flexible cartilage forms the ears and the tip of the nose, and thin layers of cartilage cushion the ends of the bones in mobile joints such as the knee and hip.

INFANT BONES

A small baby contains over 300 separate bones, many of which fuse together over the first few years of life to give the adult a total of 206 bones. The bones of a child are quite soft. Almost all children have fallen from bed – and often much further – without damage to their skeletons. In time the bone tissue begins to harden, a process that continues until the age of about 20.

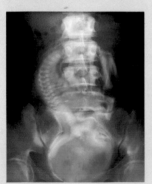

UNBORN
The bones of a child in the womb are soft and flexible.

JOINTS

The joints that connect and articulate the bones of the skeleton are its most impressive feature. There are three basic variations in the form of these joints, and some joints change their nature with age. Prominent among these are the joints between the bones that form the skull. Since the brain is well developed in the womb, the skull would be too large to pass through the birth canal if it was fully formed. Accordingly, the skull bones are not united at this stage, enabling them to collapse sufficiently to squeeze through the gap. This is why newborn babies often have oddly shaped heads. The bones come together like a jigsaw in the early months of childhood, and eventually lock solid. This form of fused jointing is called synarthrose jointing.

The opposite of this occurs in the joints of the limbs. Known as polyarthrose joints, these remain freely movable, given sufficient usage, throughout life. There are several types that allow the bones to move in different ways, and in all cases the ends of the bones are contained within a fibrous capsule containing synovial fluid, a lubricating and nourishing liquid similar in consistency to egg white. In some joints, the synovial membrane extends as a pocket called a bursa, which gives padded protection from friction where the joint's tendons lie across the bone. Strong ligaments within the capsule add strength and stability to the moving joint.

The hand, for example, is made up of 14 finger bones, five palm bones, and eight separate wrist bones. All these have movable joints to permit an unparalleled degree of flexibility. The hand is further advantaged by a highly developed sense of touch. This combination of articulation and awareness gives the hand an unrivalled ability to perform delicate, complex tasks with sublime coordination – an ability that massage skills exploit to the full.

Some joints form links between the components of protective bony structures, and many of these joints must be capable of giving way slightly under pressure. This requirement has created the third variety of joint, the amphiarthrose. In such joints a generous portion of cartilage is deposited between the ends of each bone to absorb shock and accommodate changes of shape. This arrangement allows the ribs to move where they are attached to the sternum, for easy breathing, and permits a woman's rib-cage and pelvis to accommodate the structural adaptations of pregnancy and childbirth.

THE SKELETON

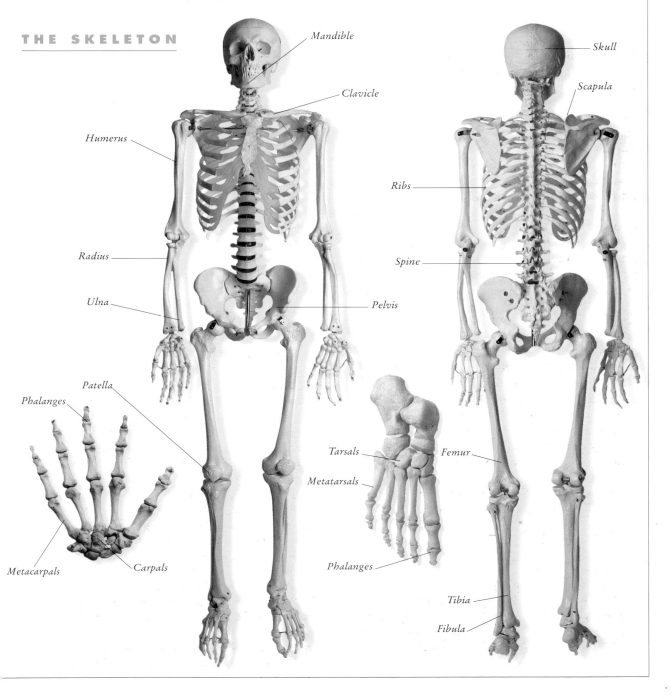

Mandible

Clavicle

Humerus

Radius

Ulna

Patella

Phalanges

Metacarpals

Carpals

Skull

Scapula

Ribs

Spine

Pelvis

Tarsals

Metatarsals

Phalanges

Femur

Tibia

Fibula

MOVABLE JOINTS

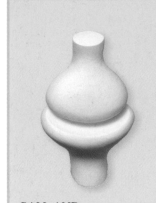
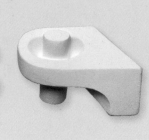
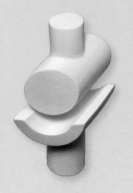

BALL AND SOCKET JOINT
The rounded head of one bone fits into a hole in another. This allows the capsule to be very loose, so the bones can be moved in almost any direction, as in the shoulder.

GLIDING JOINT
Some joints have opposing flat or slightly curved surfaces, so they glide over each other. Gliding joints have limited movement, but a chain of such joints gives good flexibility, as in the spine.

PIVOT JOINT
In a pivot joint a knob of bone rotates within a ring formed in another bone, as in the neck joint at the base of the skull. The corkscrew-like action of the lower arm is another example.

HINGE JOINT
The knee and fingers have hinge joints. A bulge on one bone fits into a hollow on another bone, and the capsule, ligaments, and tendons allow movement in one plane, like a hinge.

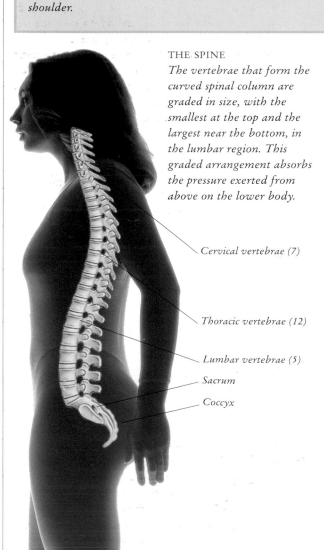

THE SPINE
The vertebrae that form the curved spinal column are graded in size, with the smallest at the top and the largest near the bottom, in the lumbar region. This graded arrangement absorbs the pressure exerted from above on the lower body.

Cervical vertebrae (7)

Thoracic vertebrae (12)

Lumbar vertebrae (5)

Sacrum

Coccyx

THE VERTEBRAL COLUMN

The spine has five major functions: it supports the weight of the head and trunk, it provides an anchor for muscle attachment, it permits movement of the back, it protects the spinal cord, and it provides a safe route for the nerves that branch off the spinal cord. Seen from the side, it has the appearance of a loaded spring, and the spinal curvature that creates this impression works in much the same way, absorbing strain and the not inconsiderable shock transmitted from the feet during walking and running.

The spine consists of a series of 26 vertebrae cushioned by intervertebral discs, arranged in a chain called the vertebral column. The individual vertebrae conform to the same basic design, but groups of vertebrae have adaptations specific to each body region. Accordingly, the vertebrae are identified and numbered from the neck downward as the cervical (7), thoracic (12), lumbar (5), sacral (5 fused), and coccygeal (3 to 4 fused). The discs which separate the vertebrae are fibro-cartilaginous, each with a tough exterior and soft, pulpy center. It is interesting to note that, regardless of the skeleton's overall height, the spinal column is roughly 25 ins/60 cm long.

Minor injuries to the postural muscles of the spine are common and relatively trivial, although they may not seem so at the time. Bone and disc disorders are more rare, and can be very serious. The cervical spine – the neck region – is relatively delicate and vulnerable to dislocation, fracture, and whiplash effects in car crashes. This is why all cars made today

BONES UNDER STRESS

The skeleton is extremely robust, but occasionally a bone may crack under stress. Such fractures are incapacitating when they occur, but if they are not complicated by other factors they heal very well – so well, in fact, that it is normally almost impossible to break the bone again in the same place. Some fractures, however, are symptoms of osteoporosis, a serious condition involving loss of bone tissue that has been linked to various factors including diet. Other skeletal problems involve the joints. Rheumatoid arthritis, for example, begins as inflammation of the connective tissue around the joint, and can cause crippling degeneration of the cartilage that cushions the joint itself. Whatever the problem, and whichever therapy is offered, bone disorders tend to respond best when treatment involves gently increasing the demands on the skeletal system as a whole.

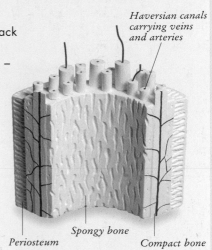

Haversian canals carrying veins and arteries

Periosteum *Spongy bone* *Compact bone*

have head restraints incorporated in the seats. The lumbar vertebrae of the lower back are very sturdy, and stress in this region is more likely to injure the discs. Under great pressure from unevenly balanced posture, the discs can herniate and spill out, causing compression on nearby spinal nerves. Under normal circumstances the coccyx is safely tucked away, but it can be damaged by an unbroken fall, and sometimes during childbirth.

LIFTING

The spine and its associated muscles are remarkably strong and resilient, but they are vulnerable to damage caused by lifting. The problem is not just a matter of trying to lift heavy objects. Olympic weightlifters can safely cope with immense weights, and there are numerous cases of ordinary people, in exceptional circumstances, raising the ends of cars or lifting logs from injured colleagues. This indicates that the context of lifting is as important as the lift itself.

Ultimately, the causes of lifting trauma can nearly always be traced to a predisposition to injury, caused by a history of previous trauma, or poor ergonomic awareness. Individual back problems therefore need individual solutions, but there are three general rules that are well worth applying, both by those who have already suffered problems and those wishing to avoid trouble.

• If you need to bend over place your feet apart and flex your knees so that your hips momentarily dip down before your spine comes upright.

• Avoid lifting any objects, or even the weight of your own upper body, when you are turned to the side – especially from the sitting position. This puts immense strain on your lumbar vertebrae, and the enormous muscle spasm you are likely to suffer is simply the body's way of protecting them.

• If you lift an object and experience a fleeting awareness that something is not quite right in your posture, do not ignore this message. Rest completely, as soon as possible, preferably in the spinal self-massage position explained on page 194.

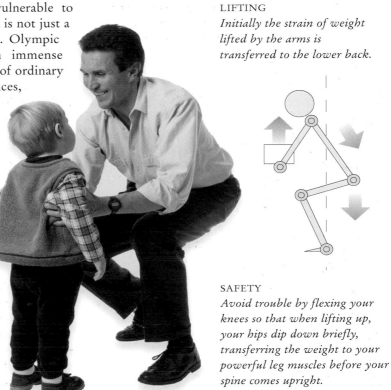

LIFTING
Initially the strain of weight lifted by the arms is transferred to the lower back.

SAFETY
Avoid trouble by flexing your knees so that when lifting up, your hips dip down briefly, transferring the weight to your powerful leg muscles before your spine comes upright.

THE MUSCLES

THE MUSCLES OF the body account for approximately 40 percent of its weight. All muscles convert chemical energy into physical power, in response to nerve signals. A muscle exerts this power by contraction, and when the nerve signal is switched off, the muscle releases and extends. Throughout the body, muscles are arranged in groups so that their contractions complement each other, and this permits a wide range of voluntary and involuntary movement. Other muscles operate alone, such as the tiny muscles that raise individual hairs in the skin in response to fear or cold.

DEPENDING ON THE particular activity they perform, muscles are structurally quite distinct. There are three basic types. Muscles that perform conscious movements, like the major limb muscles, are called voluntary or skeletal muscles. They are also known as striated (striped) muscles because the arrangement of the fibers in the muscle tissue gives it a striped appearance under the microscope. Muscles which carry out movements which require no conscious direction, like the muscles that squeeze food through the intestines, are termed involuntary muscles. On close examination, they have a smooth appearance. In a class all by itself, the cardiac muscle forms the bulk of the heart, and is responsible for pumping blood around the body with regular rhythmic contractions throughout life: an extraordinary feat of endurance.

The skeletal muscles that work your arms and legs operate under conscious control. A decision to raise an arm sends a signal through the central nervous system to trigger the contraction of the relevant muscles. These then pull on the bones to raise the arm. This freedom to improvise such actions means that the use of skeletal muscle has to be learned, and some movements can take many years to perfect. The muscles of the skeleton can also be enlarged by repetitive movements to give greater strength for strenuous activities.

The way these muscles are constructed enables them to contract very quickly, permitting the kind of explosive response that allows you to jump into the air. It also enables them to respond rapidly to reflexes – nerve signals that short-cut the brain to achieve virtually instant, involuntary action when the body is in danger. This means that skeletal muscle can in fact operate involuntarily, although you are always aware of what it is doing.

Much of the true involuntary muscle is to be found in the linings of the body's organs. Respiration, digestion, elimination, and blood circulation are achieved by involuntary muscle. The action of this smooth muscle is slow, but steady.

The instructions to the involuntary muscles are given by that part of the brain concerned with organic activity, known as the autonomic nervous system. To literally see a demonstration of the system in action, look at your eyes in a mirror and observe their

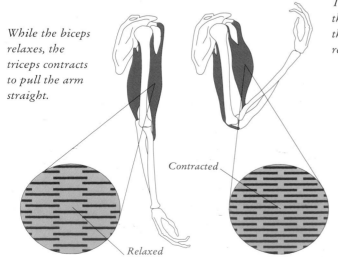

While the biceps relaxes, the triceps contracts to pull the arm straight.

The biceps flexes the arm while the triceps relaxes.

Contracted

Relaxed

MUSCLE ANTAGONISM
Muscles are almost always paired up with muscles of approximately equal strength and opposing action. The elbow is a good example. By an arrangement known as antagonism, the front muscle contracts to flex the elbow while the rear muscle relaxes. Yet the relaxation of the rear muscle is only partial. This balances the strong contraction at the front, so that, for example, when you raise a drink to your lips you are less likely to throw it over yourself.

SKELETAL MUSCLE

The mechanism of skeletal muscle contraction is well understood. Motor nerves penetrate the muscle sheath to find individual myofibrils. An electrical impulse bursts a chemical, acetycholine (ACT), on to the muscle fiber. Actin and myosin are activated and the fiber shortens. The contraction of billions of fibers results in a muscle contraction. At any point a certain number of myofibrils will be contracting, so that the muscle is not required to contract from cold. This resting state of contraction is known as muscle tone.

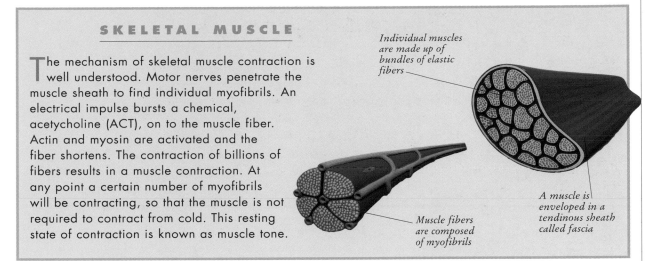

Individual muscles are made up of bundles of elastic fibers

A muscle is enveloped in a tendinous sheath called fascia

Muscle fibers are composed of myofibrils

pupil size. Place your hands over your eyes for one minute. When you remove your hands you will see that each pupil is enlarged, but then the colorful, aperture-like iris contracts the pupil to limit the amount of light entering the eye. The action is entirely involuntary.

Cardiac muscle is neurologically involuntary, yet its fibers have the striped appearance of voluntary muscles. This enables the heart to work incredibly hard, but also gives a controlled rhythm which allows a surprising amount of rest. Adding up the downtime between each of its 100,000 daily contractions, the heart is in fact at ease for approximately 20 years of a typical lifespan.

MUSCLE TONE

The nervous system maintains the muscles in a perpetual state of partial contraction in readiness for action. This state is known as muscle tone. This means that voluntary movements are not started from cold, and ensures that vital structures are always being supported by the involuntary system.

The tone of muscles is affected by emotional factors. When under the influence of fear of any kind, from mild embarrassment to terror, the involuntary nerves assume control of the whole of the muscular system as part of an autonomic response known as sympathy. This normally involves raising tone significantly, so that the skeletal muscles temporarily become ready for urgent avoiding action – "fight or flight." Meanwhile, the muscles of the organs tense up in a way that inhibits their function.

In the short term this nervous takeover may save your life, but maintained over a longer period – often through anxiety over issues that cannot easily be resolved – its usefulness is reduced. This state is now recognized in the diagnosis of stress. Its symptoms include tension of postural muscles and functional disorders such as indigestion.

The person affected by symptoms of this kind is often advised to try to relax. This is of course neurologically impossible, because the conscious plea will not be recorded by the dominant involuntary nerves.

Massage can be most helpful in this situation. The therapy involves treating the body as if the stress-making experience belonged to now – as it really does, physiologically. The massage strokes are vigorous rather than soothing, to introduce a quality of antagonism which the patient's system recognizes as validating the stress symptoms. This para-sympathy works rather like jumping over a fence to escape from danger: once the action is taken, the stress subsides.

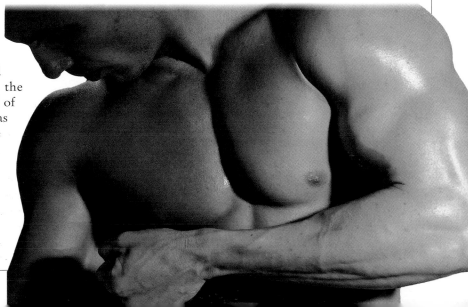

Skeletal Muscles

THE SKELETAL MUSCLES are responsible for the way the body moves. There are some 650 of these muscles, organized in complementary groups that normally act in perfect coordination to cause progressive and often powerful actions. Even minor muscle injuries can destroy the subtlety of movement by incapacitating small but vital parts of the system. Precise nervous control is also important. The involuntary muscles of the body work automatically, but control of the skeletal muscles takes years of practice to perfect.

IN ALL DESCRIPTIONS of muscles it is assumed that the body is standing facing the front: the anatomical position. Anatomists speak of moving sideways laterally, and returning to the medial line at the center. Actions in the direction of the head are cephalic, those moving behind are dorsal. This rather extravagant terminology – and the classical Greek and Latin names for individual muscles – can be daunting, but its directional basis helps to clarify how movement occurs.

The muscles are arranged around the skeleton according to functional demands. All the muscles that are responsible for backward movements are to be found behind (posterior), and those concerned with forward bending are situated to the front (anterior). However, the principle of antagonism dictates that all movements involve a sharing of muscular responsibility. Sitting down, for example, involves the posterior muscles giving a gentle rein-like tug that collapses the skeleton backwards. The anterior muscles relax only gradually, however, to ensure that this does not result in a back flip. As a result the body appears to slide down an invisible wall to reach the chair.

Convention dictates that individual muscles are distinguished in terms of origin and insertion. The part farthest away from the spine is invariably named as the insertion or pulling end. Muscles can also be described according to their shape (trapezius), number of divisions (biceps), location (tibialis), intention (levator), and direction of fiber (transversalis). The major movements of muscles are regarded as flexion when a joint is closed up, or extension when a joint is straightened out. If a limb is moved away from the body, it is abducted; if it is returned toward the body, it is adducted. There are rotator muscles and – specifically the forearm – supinators, which turn upward, and pronators, which turn down.

Muscles contract at different speeds depending on size; the larger the muscle, the lower the rate of contraction. While the arm muscle of a violinist contracts at the rate of ten per second, the speech

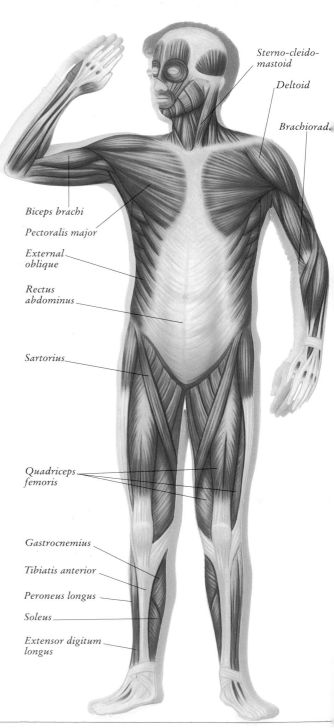

Sterno-cleido-mastoid

Deltoid

Brachiorad.

Biceps brachi

Pectoralis major

External oblique

Rectus abdominus

Sartorius

Quadriceps femoris

Gastrocnemius

Tibiatis anterior

Peroneus longus

Soleus

Extensor digitum longus

muscles of the singer she accompanies hold the body's record of 25 movements per second. The considerable heat created by all these muscle contractions is not wasted. It warms the blood, and when extra warmth is needed all the muscles join in with a spontaneous shivering.

For a full account of the muscles, you should consult a basic textbook of anatomy, but the following brief descriptions should give you a feel – in many cases literally – for the most prominent muscles you will be working on during massage. Check them out on the diagrams below.

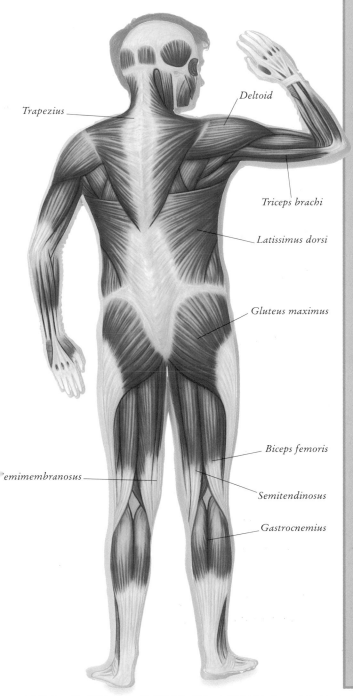

Trapezius

Deltoid

Triceps brachi

Latissimus dorsi

Gluteus maximus

Biceps femoris

emimembranosus

Semitendinosus

Gastrocnemius

THE MUSCLE GROUPS

STERNO-CLEIDO-MASTOID
These neck muscles help keep your head upright. Independently they rotate the head and flex the neck.

PECTORALIS MAJOR PECTORALIS MINOR
These draw your arm forward: feel them as you stretch across the front of your body and touch the opposite shoulder.

BICEPS BRACHI
This is the main elbow muscle, enabling you to scratch your head and offer a handshake.

BRACHIORADIALIS
This flexor and supinator twists the hand upward.

PRONATOR RADI TERES
The pronator rotates your hand downward.

FLEXOR DIGITORUM PROFUNDUS, FLEXOR CARPI RADIALIS, FLEXOR CARPI ULNARIS
Feel these finger and wrist flexors by holding your palm up and making a fist, then releasing your fingers and drawing your palm toward your elbow.

ABDOMINIS TRANSVERSALIS, RECTUS ABDOMINIS
These muscles strive to contain the abdomen. You can really feel them when you sneeze. They also help to keep the body upright.

QUADRICEPS FEMORIS
Raise the leg up in front and extend the knee to feel these working.

SARTORIUS
To feel this, the body's longest muscle, step up and rotate your thigh outward.

TIBIALIS ANTERIOR PERONEUS LONGUS
These extensors help align our footsteps.

EXTENSOR DIGITORUM LONGUS
This extensor spreads out and straightens your toes after a long day in shoes.

TRAPEZIUS
The trapezius raises your shoulders, draws them back and shortens your neck when shrugging.

DELTOID
You use this abductor muscle to draw your arm away from your body.

SCAPULARS
These are small but strong rotators that help rotate your arm in the socket of your shoulder.

TRICEPS BRACHI
The triceps is the extensor that complements the biceps. Extend your arm by your side, and the triceps will pull the arm virtually straight.

LATISSIMUS DORSI
These adductor muscles clamp your arms to your sides when surprised.

EXTERNAL OBLIQUE
From standing, reach strictly sideways down to touch the outside of your knee. You'll feel the external oblique muscle on the opposite side pull the body back up.

GLUTEALS
To feel these gluteal muscles working, balance on one leg and draw the other backward in an arabesque.

SEMITENDINOSUS, SEMIMEMBRANOSUS, BICEPS FEMORIS
These muscles assist the gluteals to extend the thigh as you walk and are the main flexors of the knees.

GASTROCNEMIUS
This flexor muscle assists the knee flexors and puts a spring in the heel for a quicker getaway.

SOLEUS
The soleus is a powerful flexor that helps its neighbor flex your ankle, pointing the foot. Stand with your toes on a book, and your heels on the ground. Raise your heels as high as possible to feel the strength of the soleus.

Muscles and Injury

ALTHOUGH THE BONES are often considered to be the armor of the body, it is really the elasticity and resilience of the muscles that protect the body from injury. If you fall over, your outstretched hand is more likely to suffer damage than the relaxed muscles of your hip or shoulder, because they absorb the shock more effectively. This shock-absorbing quality means that the muscles themselves rarely suffer incapacitating injury, yet because they are regarded as dependable, they can easily be overused and suffer from fatigue.

OVERUSE OF MUSCLES often leads to the minor injury known as strain, which is normally repaired by simply resting the muscle concerned. But muscles can be injured more severely. Exactly how severely depends on which part of the muscle is affected, and how deeply the injury affects the muscle fibers.

One potentially incapacitating injury is repetitive strain. This is a subtle disorder, and its causes are not as clear as its symptoms. We do know, however, that it afflicts those who habitually perform actions within a short range of movement. It usually affects the arms, producing pain, stiffness, and inflammation, but it

STRAIN-FREE

Repetitive strain rarely affects musicians, indicating that it is a complex condition.

does not follow the normal sequence of recovery of other forms of strain. Interestingly, musicians rarely report this condition, even though they might seem to be prime candidates for the disorder and are not without other muscle problems. It is possible that, like other puzzling muscle disorders, repetitive strain is a tonal problem caused by a combination of factors.

Muscles are aided in their locomotive responsibilities by short bands of less elastic fibers called ligaments. These bind the joints and absorb the shock of vigorous muscle contractions or unexpected movements. If the force is too great for the ligaments to contain, the result may be either a fracture to one

MASSAGE THERAPY

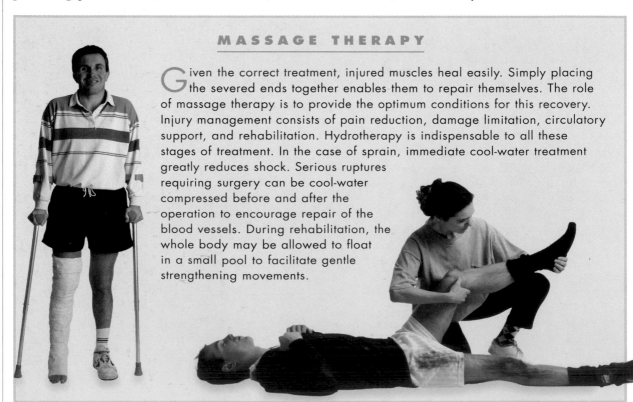

Given the correct treatment, injured muscles heal easily. Simply placing the severed ends together enables them to repair themselves. The role of massage therapy is to provide the optimum conditions for this recovery. Injury management consists of pain reduction, damage limitation, circulatory support, and rehabilitation. Hydrotherapy is indispensable to all these stages of treatment. In the case of sprain, immediate cool-water treatment greatly reduces shock. Serious ruptures requiring surgery can be cool-water compressed before and after the operation to encourage repair of the blood vessels. During rehabilitation, the whole body may be allowed to float in a small pool to facilitate gentle strengthening movements.

LOW BACK PAIN

Sufferers from low back pain often confuse their condition with the concept of the "slipped disc," but in reality the discs between the vertebrae very rarely cause back problems. Unless it is specifically caused by local trauma, low back pain is a symptom of problems with the whole posture. This is emphasized by the way sufferers from acute pain react by leaning forward until they achieve an ape-like posture, instinctively reverting to an ancestral stance in an effort to ease the spine.

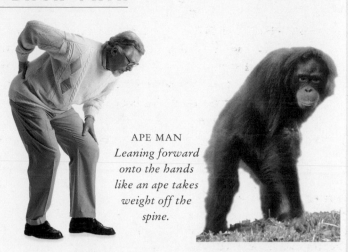

APE MAN
Leaning forward onto the hands like an ape takes weight off the spine.

or more of the joint's bones, or a tearing of the ligaments called a sprain. This generally occurs at either the ankle or the wrist, and conventional therapy involves encasing the joint in plaster to immobilize it while it heals.

The rarest form of damage, given the pliability of muscle tissue, is a tear of the muscle fibers. This type of injury typically affects the end of a muscle where the fibers are concentrated to form the tendon. Most at risk are athletes such as soccer players, and people involved in violent impacts who sustain excessive stretch or a direct blow on the muscle concerned. Such damage usually requires surgery to reattach the torn tissues.

A less dramatic form of tear is called a rupture, in which the fibers of the muscle are incompletely torn and often spill out from the enclosing sheath of the muscle. A variant of this affects the abdominal muscle, although in this case it is the small intestine that protrudes through the gap. Such ruptures often occur at the junction of the abdomen and thigh, where there is a structural weak point. The condition sounds alarming, but it can be safely self-managed unless it becomes serious or is irritated by strenuous activities such as sports.

Muscles need rest if they are to renew themselves. This is normally achieved not only by sleep but by recreation, which brings different sets of muscles into play. If muscles do not get sufficient rest, they can become irritated. The evidence for this is the knots which are found during massage, otherwise known as fibrositis. This condition can also suggest emotional strains, especially since fibrositis is commonly found in the shoulder area. During massage it is not unusual for a patient to verbalize the tension found in the neck and shoulder with comments such as, "Ouch, this is really painful, but it feels good, go deeper!"

MUSCLE CRAMP

During strenuous exercise, the normal processes of breathing and circulation provide the muscles with oxygen and blood sugar for energy, and eliminate accumulated acidic waste products. If these processes are inadequate, a muscle may contract protectively to await supplies before continuing further work, the condition known as cramp. It is not possible or even desirable to override this involuntary defensive measure. Locally, cramp is best relieved by rest and increased respiration. This should be followed by careful and gradual stretching of the muscle involved, accompanied by effleurage. If cramp occurs regularly during normal, non-strenuous activity, or in bed, this suggests poor muscle tone, which is best remedied by attention to diet and stress levels, coupled with massage therapy.

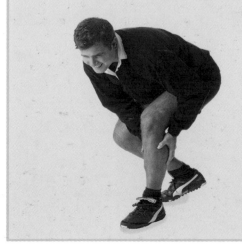

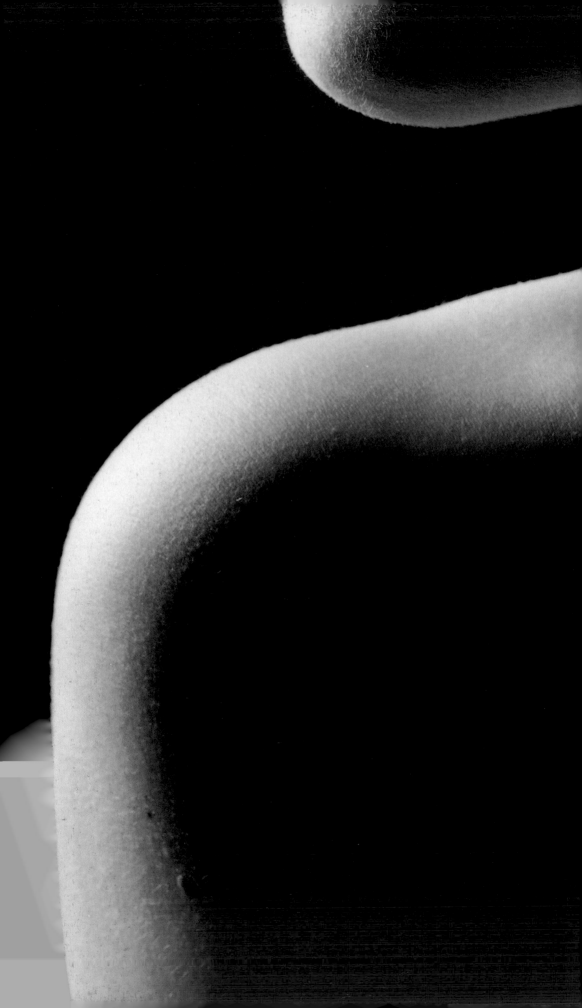

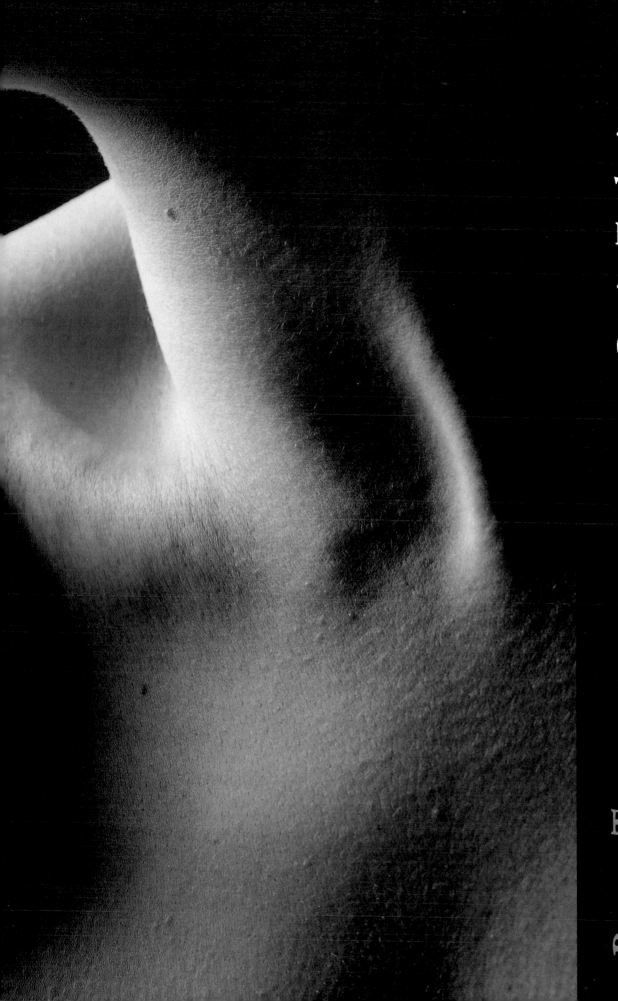

Basic Techniques

PART THREE

THE TECHNIQUES

THE ESTABLISHMENT of massage therapy in Europe, if not throughout the world, stems from the work of Swedish professor Pier Heidrich Ling. Ling devised a classic formula for *effleurage, petrissage,* and *percussion,* as shown opposite, combined with *mobilizing* movements. Although he was not trained in conventional medicine,

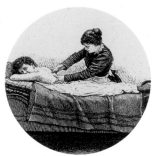

Massage was a common therapy in nineteenth-century Europe.

Ling was able to carry out studies on ill and injured patients that showed the direct physiological and psychological benefits of the individual massage strokes. Ling's clear descriptions of massage enabled budding practitioners to visualize the purpose of the strokes, and his work has become the basis of effective massage treatment today.

FLEXIBILITY FOR MASSAGE

To prepare your hands and wrists for giving massage, try this flexibility exercise. Only about one in ten achieve the full movement at their first attempt, because it is both difficult and rather confusing! The exercise can also be done after massaging to loosen up the tension caused by overworking your hands.

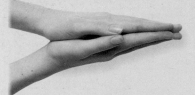

1 Loosen your arms and extend them a little. Place your hands flat against one another, exactly aligned from heel to fingertip.

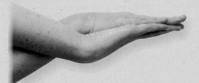

2 Cross your wrists, left over right, and replace the hands together. You will begin to feel your wrists stretching.

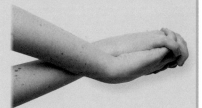

3 Fully interlock your fingers, but take care not to clench them too tightly.

4 Straighten your elbows and open out your hands by raising your left arm. Remember to keep the fingerlock loose.

5 Fully flex your elbows at shoulder height. Your hands may feel that they are being wrung out, and if so this may be far enough for the first attempt. To reach full stretch, drop your right elbow as far as possible and extend the left arm slowly. Straighten both arms. Reverse the action to undo, and effleurage from the fingertips to the forearms before repeating the exercise with right hand over left.

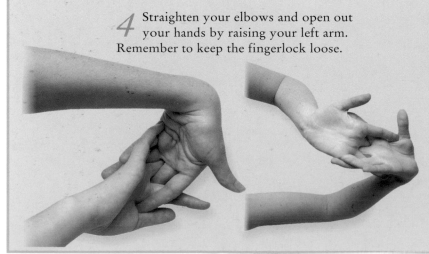

LING'S MOVEMENTS

Massage is given in a flowing sequence, in which one stroke blends seamlessly with another. This classic formula for massage shows the strokes needed to give an effective treatment. The vital transition between the pressure strokes is provided by effleurage, which also introduces and concludes the massage.

EFFLEURAGE
Concluding   Introductory

PERCUSSION
Stimulation

MOBILIZATION

PETRISSAGE
SUPERFICIAL STROKES
Pressure

EFFLEURAGE
Draining

EFFLEURAGE

For effleurage, lay your hands across the patient's body with fingers together and thumbs slightly stretched. Stroke smoothly, initially without pressure, following the contours of the body. Smooth the skin in the direction of the heart after petrissage strokes.

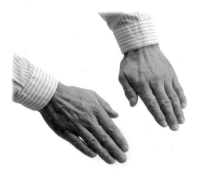

CIRCLING

FANNING

LIGHT PRESSING

FRICTION

PETRISSAGE
AND KNEADING

For kneading, use the whole hand, with fingers together and thumbs outstretched, to squeeze the rounder contours of the body. Petrissage is a lighter squeezing action, using only the thumbs and fingertips to work on slimmer or flatter muscles.

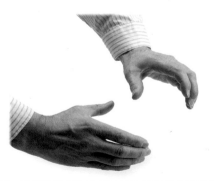

DEEP PRESSING

PUMMELING

STRETCHING

ROLLING

RAKING

THUMBING

PERCUSSION

Apply percussion by lightly striking the body using different parts of your hands, keeping your wrists loose. Begin slowly, increase to moderate speed, then build to a crescendo before stopping abruptly.

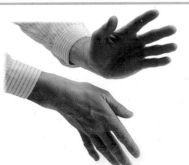

HACKING

CUPPING

BEATING

TAPPING

PICKING UP

EFFLEURAGE

EFFLEURAGE IS THE preparatory and concluding stroke of massage. It feels soothing, especially for slender patients, while gently bringing awareness to the part of the body being treated. Effleurage is noninvasive, since it puts no pressure on the body and does not attempt to move it. Although very superficial in comparison with other strokes, effleurage is profound in its effects. This is because of the way its influence penetrates the skin and feeds back to the brain through the peripheral nerves. Effleurage also helps attune the massager to the patient and is a good discipline for those who tend to rush into deeper strokes prematurely.

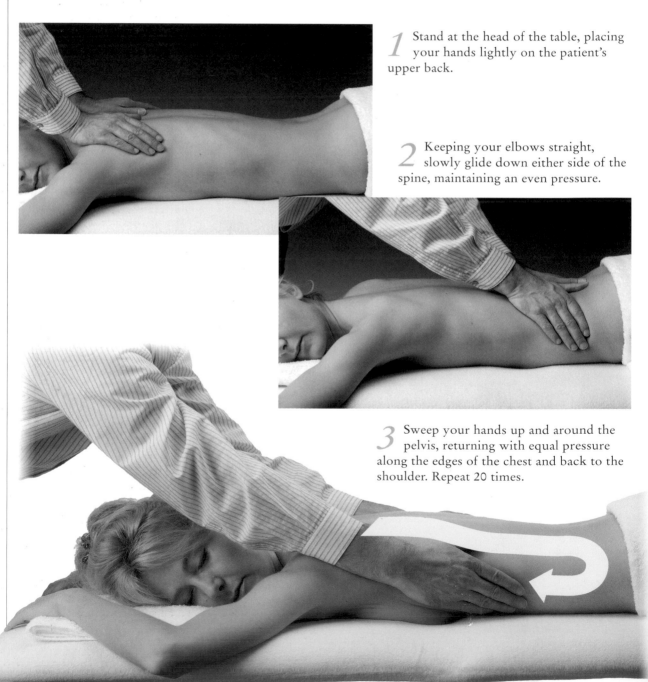

1 Stand at the head of the table, placing your hands lightly on the patient's upper back.

2 Keeping your elbows straight, slowly glide down either side of the spine, maintaining an even pressure.

3 Sweep your hands up and around the pelvis, returning with equal pressure along the edges of the chest and back to the shoulder. Repeat 20 times.

Effleurage of the Face

NOT ONLY DOES effleurage alone provide a virtually complete massage for the face, but its extended effect may be felt throughout the body. Indeed, spontaneous "face-washing" stroking can be observed in someone attempting to dispel uncomfortable tension. This works because the peripheral nerves of the face are intimately connected with deeper nervous controls that modify rising pressures in the body and return the system to a calmer state after excitement.

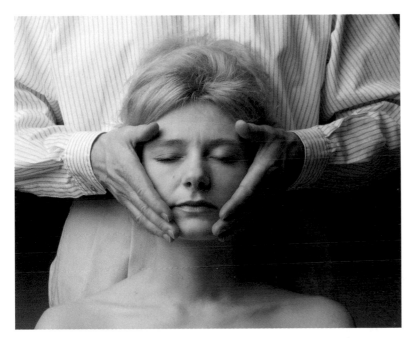

1 Ask your patient to rest her head against your abdomen. Then place your outstretched hands against the sides of her face and effleurage toward the ears.

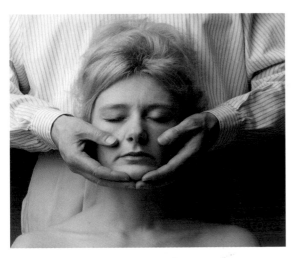

2 Support the chin lightly and effleurage by drawing the edges of your thumbs from the cheekbones to the jaw.

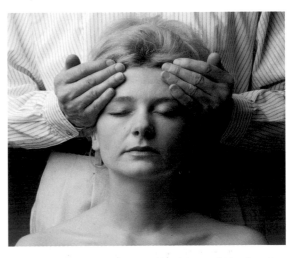

3 Place your hands on the front of the head, with the fingertips meeting. Smoothly effleurage from the forehead to the temples and continue into the hair, right around the head.

KNEADING

OST PEOPLE ASSOCIATE massage with the deepest stroke, known as kneading, where curved muscles such as those on the front of the thigh are squeezed with the whole hand and thumb. This stroke breaks down deep tensions and conditions muscles so they have even tone. It encourages the muscles to be more sponge-like, and this helps local circulation and assists the heart. The experience of being kneaded can be very emotional. As deep tensions are released, groans of delight can sometimes give way to tears.

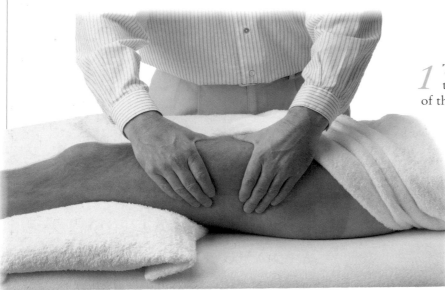

THE LEG

1 The front of the thigh is one of the most heavily muscled areas of the entire body, and responds well to kneading. Ensure that the knee is well pillowed to encourage the release of deep tension, especially with male patients because of their slightly different thigh angle. Grasp the middle of the front of the leg with open hands, not tightly, but so there is no space between hand and leg.

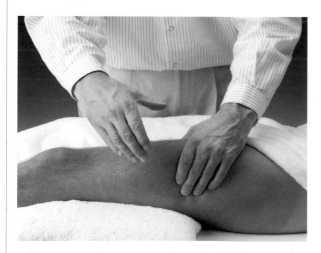

2 Release your grip on the thigh and, as you do so, press into the muscle with the other hand. Increase your grip with a sponge-like action, but do not squeeze with your fingertips.

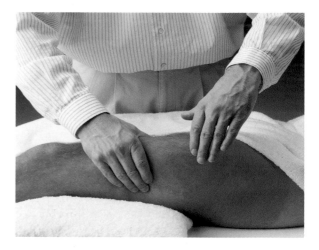

3 Release the muscle for the other hand to take control and repeat, making the stroke as identical as possible. Work up and down the thigh, varying your grip according to the shape of the muscle toward the knee or front of the pelvis.

KNEADING OTHER AREAS

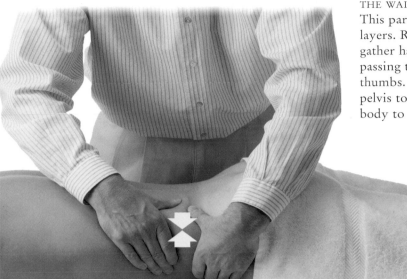

THE WAIST

This part of the body contains deep muscle layers. Reach over the couch and attempt to gather handfuls of waist, drawing them in and passing them between your hands and thumbs. Move your hands up and down from pelvis to rib-cage and from the edge of the body to the spine.

PRECAUTION

Kneading can be overdone, and both the therapist and patient can become exhausted. To prevent this, regularly intersperse the kneading strokes with effleurage.

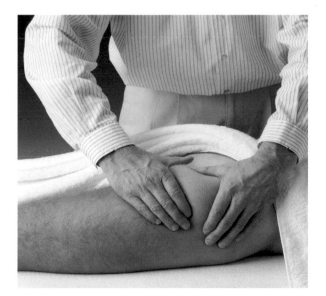

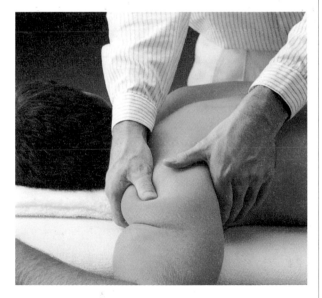

BUTTOCKS

The round muscle layers of the buttock fit into the pelvis rather like the layers of a large onion. To massage these muscles thoroughly you will need to apply deep pressing strokes, using the whole of your hand. The largest nerve of the body passes through the buttock, so avoid pinching it or the leg will become more tense than relaxed.

TOP OF THE ARM

The muscle at the top of the arm, near the shoulder, is large enough to benefit from kneading. Hold it between your hands so that it can be squeezed, while at the same time sustaining strong thumb pressure.

PETRISSAGE

THE STROKE KNOWN as petrissage involves taking hold of the edge of a muscle, or a part of the muscle that lies close to the bone, and squeezing it with fingertips and thumbs. This stroke is most suitable for the sinewy muscles in the limbs and upper back. It aims to adjust tension rather than force it out, since force would be resisted by this kind of muscle. Petrissage allows detailed work on the body and is recommended for children and older adults. Giving petrissage also benefits the massager, since it develops finger sensitivity.

THE LEG

1 With a generous pillow placed under the knee, hold the groin muscles between your fingertips and thumb, leaving a space between the palms and the leg. Start the stroke just below the knee with your fingers well under the leg, using only moderate pressure.

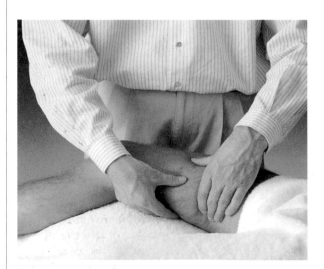

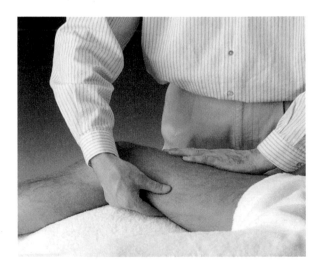

2 Move your hands slowly along the groin muscle, squeezing rhythmically with alternate pressures that get lighter toward the upper leg. When you are two-thirds of the way along the leg, return toward the knee, steadily increasing the pressure as you go.

3 Optionally, steady the leg with one hand and use the other to petrissage progressively up and down the groin muscle. Such single hand strokes are more focused but seem to take more energy, perhaps because they are less rhythmic.

PETRISSAGE OF THE BACK

RIDGE OF THE SHOULDER
The classic massage stroke, this makes practitioners wince when misrepresented in films. It is a deep movement, done mainly by the ball of your thumb as you work along the shoulder with your fingers lightly resting on the top.

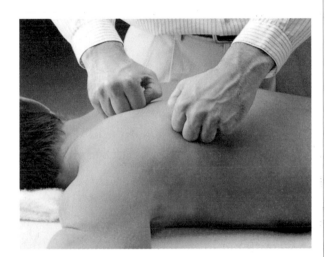

SCAPULA
Treat the slender muscles of the back with knuckling petrissage. Use small, middle, or great knuckles to suit the muscle. In all cases drag your knuckles erratically across the scapulas and the space between them.

ALTERNATIVE SCAPULA
With lightweight patients you can employ the same basic technique as knuckling petrissage but using rigid fingers instead of – or as well as – your knuckles. Drag them over the scapula in a similar way.

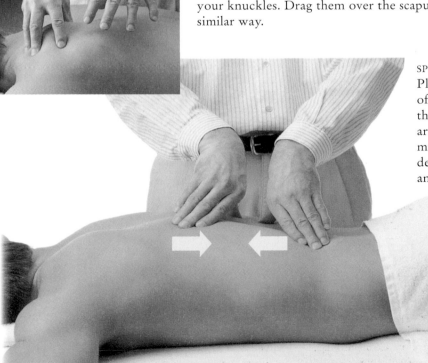

SPINE
Place your fingertips on one side of the spine and your thumbs on the other. In this position they are resting over the erector muscles of the back. Lightly depress your fingers and thumbs and slide them back and forth toward each other, up and down the back. This stroke should be done toward the end of a back massage, since the erectors belong to the deepest muscle layer.

SUPERFICIAL STROKES

THE SUPERFICIAL STROKES are a series of movements derived from petrissage. They are superficial because they are only skin deep, yet their effects can be profound. This is because they treat the skin as an organ, interacting with its nerves and circulation to provide benefits throughout the body. Superficial strokes are ideal for oil massage and injury treatments. In aromatherapy they provide a light but stimulating movement and just enough contact for oily hands. For injury massage, they loosen the tissues, increase circulation, and relieve painful pressures.

Circling

CIRCLING IS A SWEEPING stroke, like an effleurage that lightly drags over the skin. The whole of the back can be circled in any direction, in small or large movements. The stroke can also be used over the buttocks, increasing in depth to grade into the stroke known as pressing. It is very effective when used as a warming introductory stroke to a full back massage. Miniature circling can be applied with the fingertips held closely together.

1 Take up a steady stance close to the couch. Lean across the patient's back and place a reinforced hand on the side of her waist. Make a good skin contact.

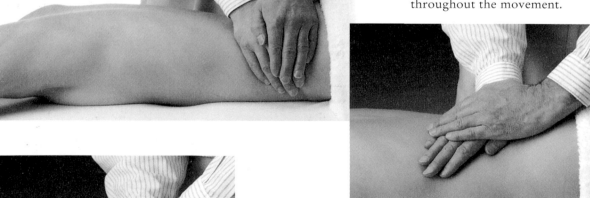

2 Begin to sweep your hands up toward her rib-cage by rotating your wrists. Try to maintain even pressure throughout the movement.

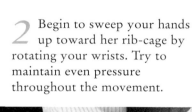

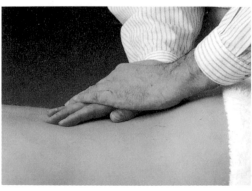

3 Continue the wrist movement until you reach the other side of the waist, then push smoothly over to complete the circle. Repeat the circles, increasing their depth slightly until you create some warmth between hand and skin.

Fanning

FANNING IS A COMBINATION of friction and stretching. It is effective over broad areas of muscles, such as those found in the abdomen and upper back. It consists of a steady, repetitive pressure, spreading evenly across the body with fingers trailing at a light stretch. Done briskly, it is a suitable preparation for aromatherapy back massage. It is also a very soothing, almost hypnotic stroke if done slowly at the conclusion of massage in place of effleurage.

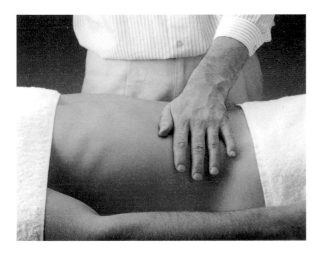

1 Standing to the patient's left side, extend your arm and place the heel of your left hand in the center of his abdomen, with your fingers laid over his waist.

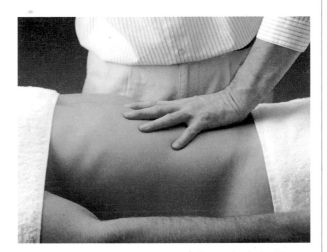

2 Make an upper fanning stroke by rotating your hand toward his ribs, swinging your elbow in the direction of his feet. Focus the movement in the heel of your hand and allow your fingers to trail passively. Continue over until your fingertips reach the nearside of his waist, by which time your elbow will point away from his body.

3 Replace your left hand with your right hand, placing it a little higher on the patient's abdomen. Complete a lower fan by rotating your hand smoothly back to the patient's waist on the far side.

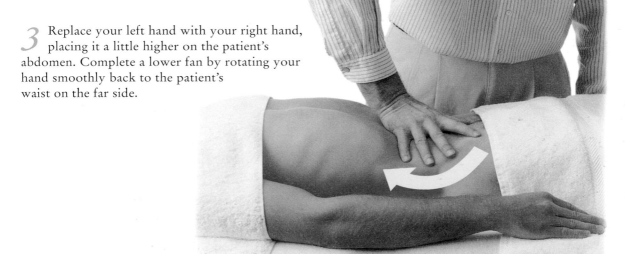

Rolling

ROLLING IS VERY good conditioning for the skin, toning it and increasing its circulation and drainage. Used toward the end of a treatment, it is a good indication of the success of the previous strokes. If all is well, the skin should be warm and supple, and rolling over the deeper structures should not cause pain. If some tightness is felt, the area should be raked over or given repeat thumbing.

1 Place your hands across the shoulder area. Gather the skin between the fingers and thumb of both hands and hold gently.

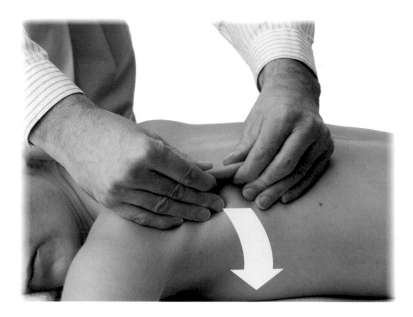

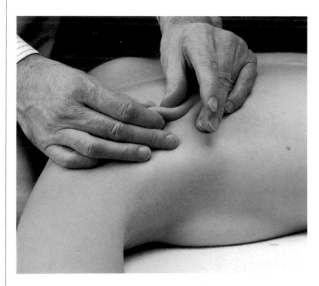

2 Walk your hands forward a few fingers, increasing to a slight stretching pressure on the skin. Slide your thumb toward your fingers to create a wavelike motion.

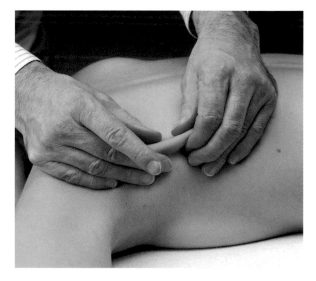

3 Continue walking your fingers and pushing gently with both thumbs, until the original wave in the skin is taken to the edge of the chest. Repeat all over the back, working from the spine toward the edge of the body, then from upper to lower back.

Picking up

*PICKING UP IS a short, tugging stroke used over broad areas for a tonal effect.
It has no similarity to the holding quality of kneading, since whatever tissue can
be picked up between the fingers is immediately allowed to spring back.
It is aimed at the skin, but it also achieves a reaction from muscles that stretch
across areas of the body, such as the abdominal muscles and the smaller structures
associated with the shoulder blade.*

1 Put a pillow beneath the patient's knees.
Place your fingertips and thumb on the
center of the abdomen. Keep your arms steady.

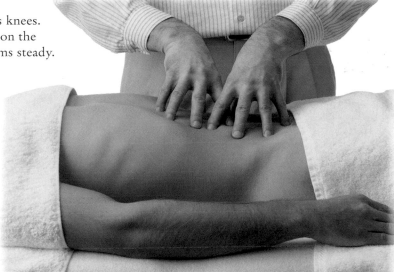

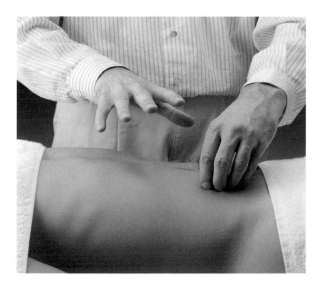

2 Press inward gently with your left hand and
quickly contract the fingers, while at the same
time lifting and spreading the fingers of your right
hand. Aim to achieve the snatching effect without
pinching the patient's skin.

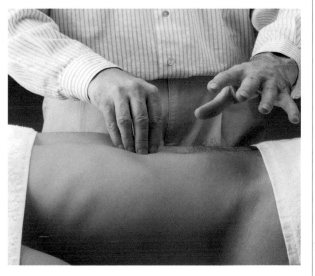

3 Reverse the action, snatching at the abdomen
with the fingers of your right hand while
spreading your left hand. Increase speed and
depth, working in bursts of 20 seconds.

Friction

FRICTION STROKES MAY be the "rubbing" spoken of by Hippocrates in his description of massage. The intention of friction is not only to warm up an area, but to gently tug the layers of skin, fascia, and muscle to achieve a loosening effect. This is most often required after an injury, where a complication has produced adhesion. Accelerated friction can also have a vibrating effect on tired muscles that are too painful to be squeezed. By making firm contact during friction, the stroke is converted into the stroke known as "shaking."

1 Place the edges of your hands parallel across the back of the thigh. Make a good skin contact but do not press down. If the legs are hairy, take the precaution of using a little talc or oil.

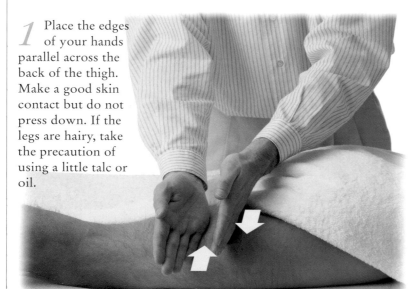

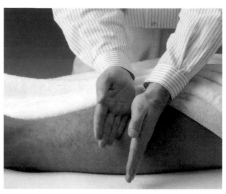

2 Move up and down the thigh, quickly sliding your hands backward and forward in short bursts of 20 seconds or so. The stroke should produce some heat, but be careful not to overdo the effect.

FRICTION USED ON OTHER AREAS

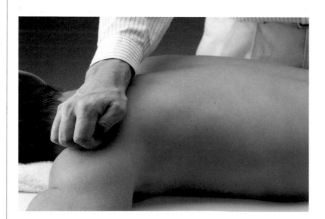

UPPER SHOULDER
Make a loose fist, turn the small knuckles onto the shoulder area and make skin contact. Using a side-to-side wrist action, make wavy frictions in all directions.

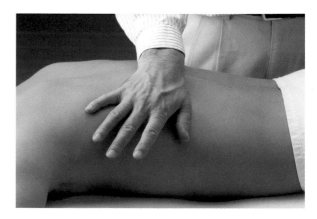

CHEST AND RIBS
Extend your fingers so they spread out a little and make contact against the side of the chest. Using similar but more exaggerated wrist movements, rub up and down along the whole of the rib-cage.

Raking

SOMETIMES CALLED "clawing" or "ruffling feathers," this is a vigorous stroke that feels a lot more relaxing than it looks. One reason for this is that the initial, superficial stimulation of raking is converted into a sensation of containment as the skin firms up under the strokes. It can be done as the first, warming stroke of a back massage, or used over a muscle that is locked in spasm. Raking is particularly useful in the rehabilitation stage of injury, as a means of raising awareness before exercise.

1 Raise your hands right up on to their fingertips, thumb included. Place them lightly on the patient's body, slightly apart but close enough to be working on the same area.

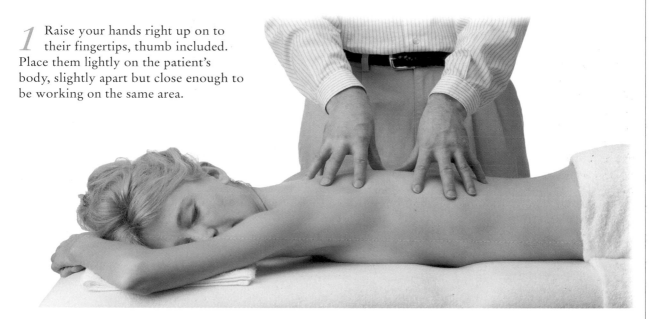

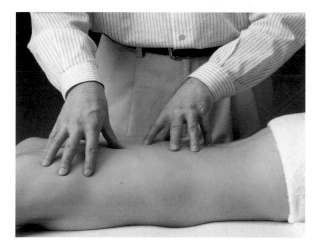

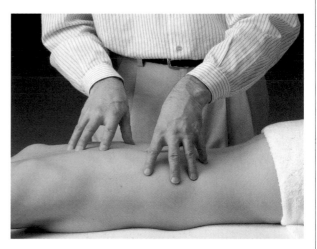

2 Draw your hands briskly past each other, keeping your wrists tight. Rake your fingers backward and forward across the patient's body 10 times.

3 Move to another area, repeating the action, until you have treated the whole back. The space between the scapulas is particularly responsive to this raking stroke.

Pummeling

PUMMELING INVOLVES holding your hands against the patient's body and shaking them to achieve deep vibration of the muscles and other structures within. The areas of the body that benefit most from this stroke are the legs and shoulders, where it is not possible to use the picking-up stroke on the muscles. To perform the stroke properly you must take care not to lift your hands and break contact with the skin, since this would transform the pummeling, shaking effect into a form of percussion.

1 Reach over and place the edges of your fists against the outside of the thigh. Stand close to the couch and focus the stroke in your hands by slightly locking your elbows.

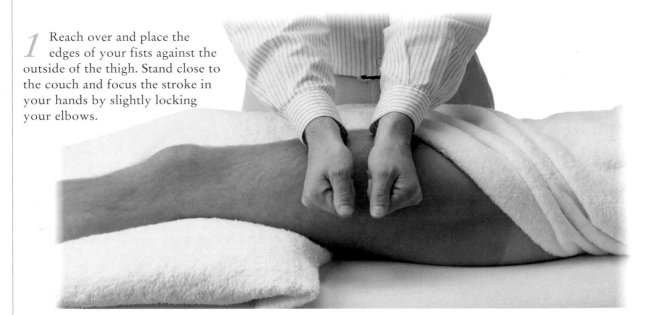

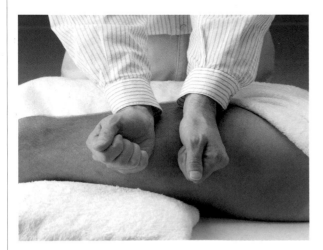

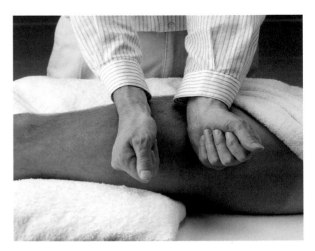

2 Roll back your right hand a little from the wrist, while steadying your left hand. Return your right hand to the start position, and at the same time roll back the left.

3 Increase speed until you achieve a forward and backward rolling action. Remember to keep your elbows extended and maintain pummeling at full speed for 10 seconds. The action exerts a pressure deep within the leg without actually striking it.

Thumbing

THUMBING IS A twisting of the skin over a tight or adhering muscle. It is very specific and allows movement over a tense area without discomfort. Such tension often appears as a small reddening of the skin after effleurage and this is an indication for thumbing. If the stroke is given with the hands flat and further apart, it can be used over a larger area of the body. The thumbs should be kept straight and spun across the skin, making a slight indentation.

1 Place your fingertips and thumbs on the patient's upper back, with your fingers drawn together and thumbs slightly apart. Keep your wrists steady.

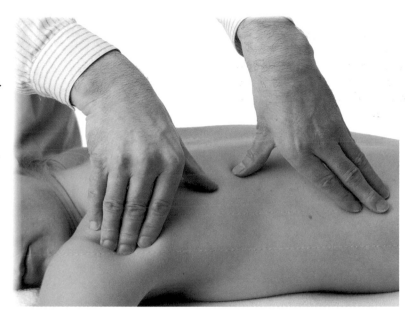

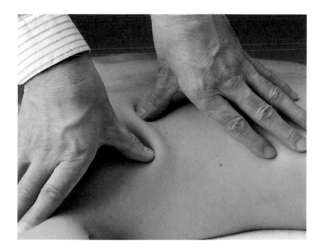

2 Depress your hands to make firm contact and move them so your left thumb slides behind your right in a small semicircle, while at the same time your right thumb slides in front of your left.

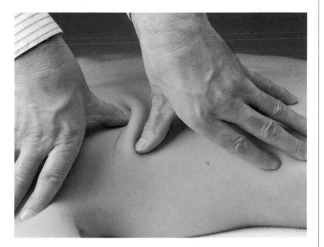

3 Repeat in reverse and increase speed, making S-shaped sliding movements on the skin. Maintain for 20 seconds and then repeat, changing the angle of your hands in the first position.

Stretching

THE SKIN IS NOT just a passive membrane clothing the body; it is an elastic, muscular organ that helps contain the muscles. The elasticity and resilience of the skin and its muscles is demonstrated by the way it recovers from pregnancy, but it benefits from stretching strokes, which exercise the skin and keep it moving freely over the structures beneath it. Because of shared nervous controls, organs such as the lungs can be influenced by treating the overlying skin.

1 Place both your hands side by side on the patient's back, palm down. Take up a firm contact.

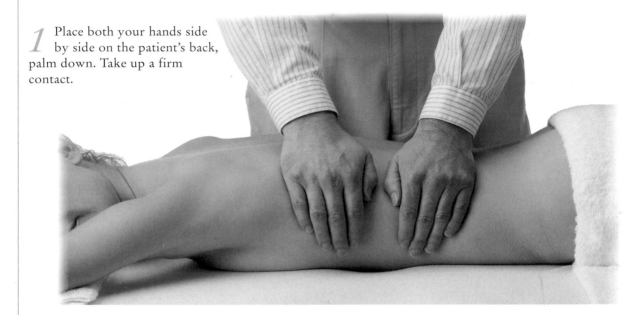

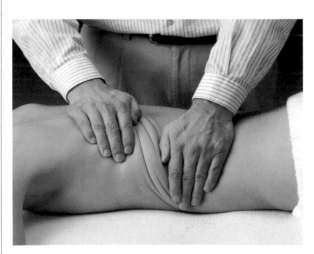

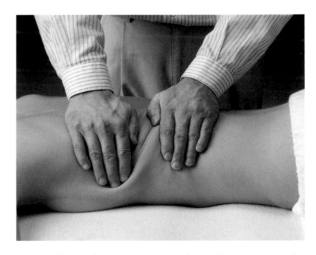

2 Press on the back and slowly slide your hands in opposite directions, moving the skin as much as possible. You may not move it far, but even a little is enough to begin with.

3 Release the pressure, but keep in contact and perform the movement in reverse. Repeat this push-slide, push-slide six times, then move up and across to treat the entire back.

Pressing

THIS FORM OF pressing involves a push-slide movement with the hands held in a crossover position to ensure even pressure. It is particularly suitable for the center and edges of the back, and in passing it provides a convenient and useful kidney friction. Avoid direct contact with the spine at the waist or the base of the neck but the chest can be firmly pressed. For comfort, the patient should exhale at the pressure of the first position and inhale on the return stroke.

1 Place your hands together, with wrists crossed over, on the lower back. Take up contact with the heels of your hands, which should rest to the side of the spine on each side.

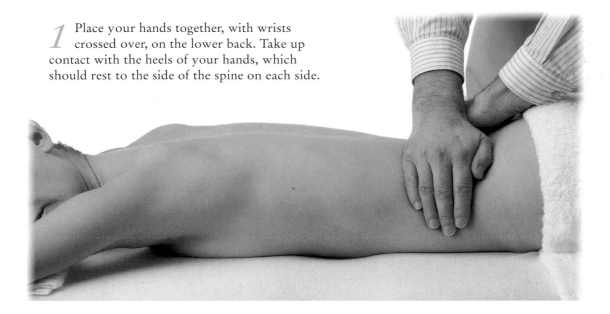

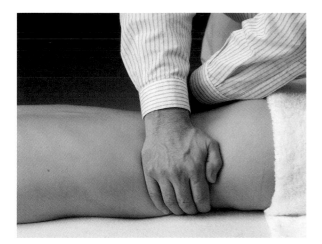

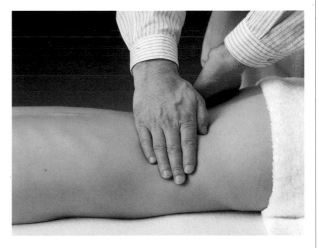

2 Push and slide each hand off-center and compress around the patient's waist. Pause to check that the stroke is synchronized with the patient's breathing.

3 Draw your hands tighter against the body and return to center with a moderate pressure. Repeat twice more, then advance a little way up the back and continue the movements up to the level of the shoulders.

PERCUSSION

MASSAGE TREATMENT is completed by the stimulating strokes of percussion. These are designed to reintegrate the body so that the patient's transition from deep relaxation back to everyday movement is complete. Percussion involves striking the muscles and skin using a variety of unusual wrist movements. Contact is made with different parts of the hand depending on the part of the body being treated. The reintegration is achieved by percussing slowly at first, gradually building up speed to a crescendo, then stopping abruptly after approximately 20 seconds.

Hacking

HACKING IS A sympathetic wake up call to the muscles, which can be applied to every part of the body except the face. The technique has been made familiar by media representations of massage, but it is actually quite difficult to do well. The main challenge involved in this stroke – and in other percussions – is striking evenly with both hands: a skill that comes naturally with practice.

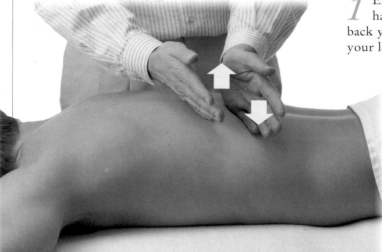

1 Extend your wrists and fingers and lay your hands parallel across the patient's back. Flick back your right hand and incline the fingers of your left hand to the body, from the wrists alone.

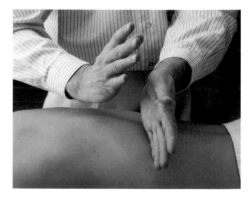

2 Quickly reverse this movement so that your hands pass by each other, and repeat the action continuously at moderate speed.

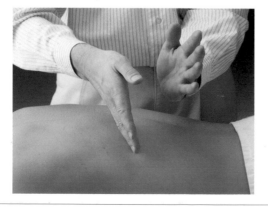

3 Once you have established a rhythm, lighten up the stroke as if shaking your hands against the patient's body. Keep your fingers parallel but relaxed; as you work you should hear them striking against one another.

Cupping

CUPPING PREPARES THE larger muscle groups for activity after massage. It is used most frequently on the rounder contours of the body, but it can also be used over the rib-cage to loosen respiratory congestion. The cup that you make with your hands should feel watertight, and the wrists perform the same type of controlled flicking movement used in hacking. You will hear a deep hollow sound as the air is beaten from the surface of the skin. Red finger marks reveal that the cupping is too shallow, so if this occurs, begin again with more tension in your palms.

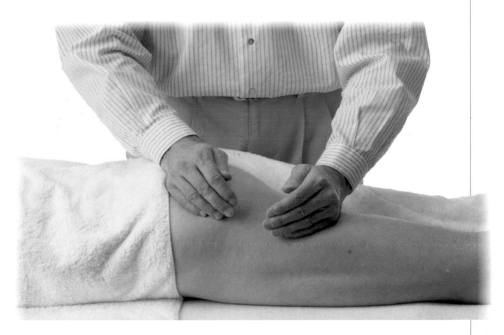

1 Look into your hands and make cups that would be tight enough to contain water. Keep each thumb straight and close to the index finger. Turn your hands over and place them both palm down on the patient's buttock.

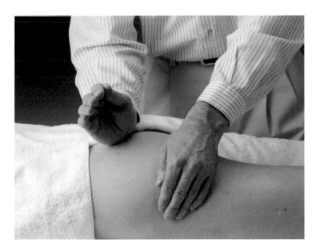

2 Contract your wrist to flick your right hand back from the patient's body and incline the other hand toward the buttock, moving them only from the wrists.

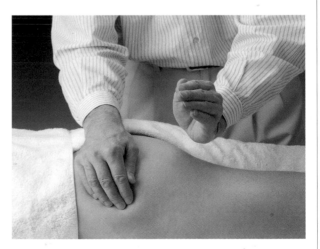

3 Alternate your hands, striking the patient's body quite sharply, then soften the stroke by shaking your hands against the body. Cupping should make a loud popping sound as each cupped hand strikes the skin.

Beating

BEATING IS THE most appropriate form of percussion for the strongly muscled areas of the body, and for people who are generally well-muscled. It is the deepest, most penetrating of the percussion strokes, and aims to stimulate right through all the muscle layers. The large muscles of the buttocks, upper arms, and legs all benefit from this treatment. Your hands should remain tense throughout the stroke, since, as with other forms of percussion, all the action is generated by movement of the wrist.

1 Make tight fists with your hands, extend your wrists, and place both clenched fists lightly on the front of the patient's thigh.

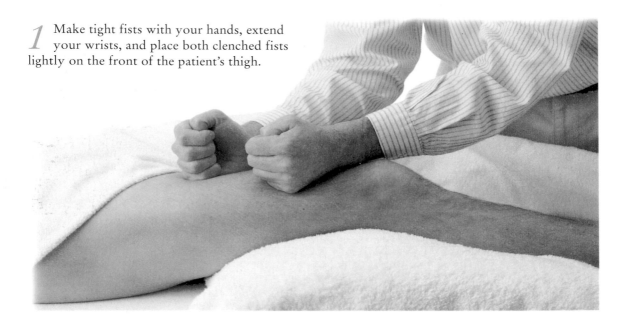

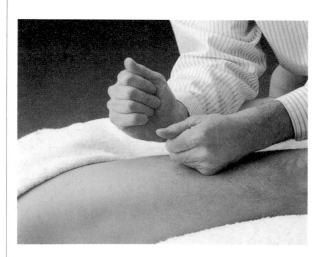

2 Flick your right hand back while inclining your left hand to the leg. Then beat your right hand on to the leg as you withdraw your left hand.

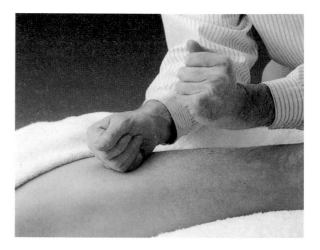

3 Continue, picking up speed and rhythm. Beating can be quite strenuous, so 10 seconds may be sufficient. Be careful not to strike any large bones nearby, since this will jar the skeleton.

Tapotement

VARIOUS TAPPING movements – known as tapotement – can be applied to the face and any other areas that, for any reason, are in a delicate state. This is the most superficial form of percussion, but it can often be carried out with the greatest speed. Tapotement of the face is locally stimulating but generally relaxing, owing to the reflex reaction that any touching of the face triggers in the vagus nerve. This means that the tapotement stroke makes an ideal conclusion to a facial massage.

1 Hold your hands lightly open and bring your fingers into contact with the underside of the chin, flicking upward all along the jaw line. Maintain a steady, moderate speed for 20 seconds.

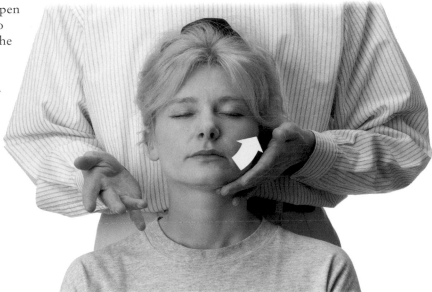

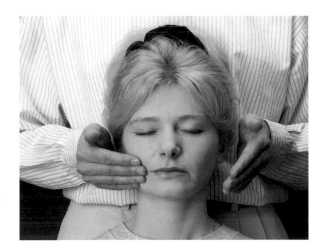

2 With your fingers held together, tap the cheeks lightly by flexing your knuckles alternately. You can extend this stroke to the temples and forehead, but apply it much more lightly. The whole contact should last roughly 20 seconds.

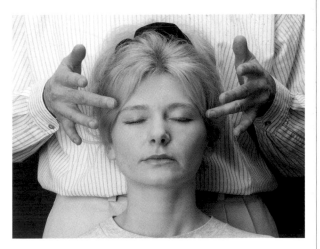

3 Drum your fingertips lightly and slowly all over the face, then with increased speed for 20 seconds. Avoid contact with the eyes and tip of the nose but do not exclude the ears, since these normally enjoy the experience.

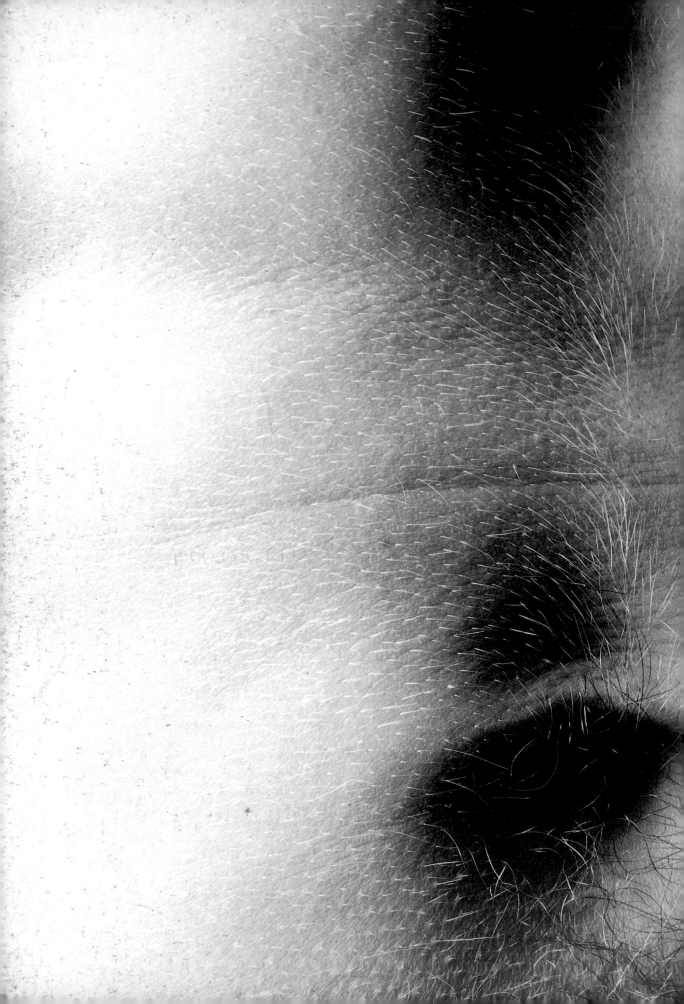

PART FOUR

PREPARING FOR MASSAGE

MASSAGE TAKES place everywhere – from smart health farms to street corners in India; in the day room of a home for the elderly and in the delivery room of the maternity unit. Sometimes the circumstances are dictated by necessity, such as in a stadium when an athlete's muscles have seized up, but the ideal setting is more relaxed, in tune with the aims and methods of massage. Some settings, such as by the sea, facilitate massage because they reflect the sensual atmosphere of effleurage. Taking care to work in the right conditions will also help to maintain the physical health of the massager.

EQUIPMENT

TOWELS
Keep fresh towels in the sunlight or on a heater to warm them up in preparation for treatment.
Keep a stack of extra towels in a convenient place in case the patient becomes cold at any point.

TABLE OR FLOOR?
Working on the floor, with a futon mattress, has the advantage of simplicity. However, it makes the more active techniques difficult and even potentially damaging to the massager.

BEYOND A PAIR of sensitive hands, the equipment needed for massage depends very much on the type of practice being offered. In the larger cities, itinerant massage practitioners are to be found in offices, attending to workers at their desks. More thorough massage may demand some very practical hardware, such as a portable treatment couch for home visits. Other styles of therapy may involve soft furnishings, screened-off areas, low lighting, and background music to create a soothing atmosphere.

FLOOR, COUCH, OR TABLE?

The first requirement is something for the patient to lie on. Whether you give massage on the floor, on a converted dining table, or on an electrically operated treatment couch is a matter of style and finance. The simplicity of the shiatsu setting, consisting of a plain futon mattress and very little else, obviously involves minimal expense. This approach can be very effective psychologically, although working on the floor cannot be recommended for the more active massage techniques. Meanwhile, the technological approach, which might involve adjustable couches, heat lamps, and gyrating accoutrements, requires a major investment, although it will probably impress some potential patients.

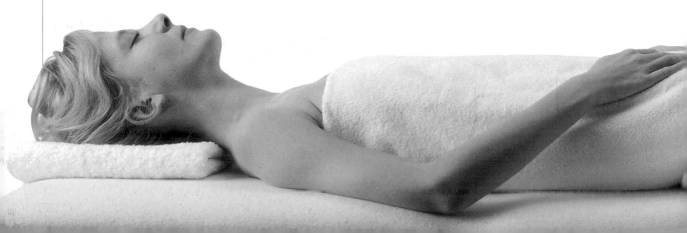

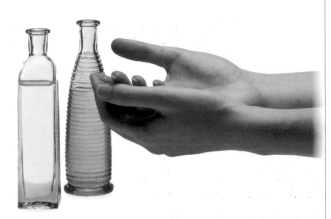

Initially, it is best to make use of the facilities you have to hand. Many illustrious careers in massage therapy originated on reconstructed dining furniture. The obvious problem to overcome with a dining room table is lack of length, but this is easily rectified by placing large pillows at the end so the patient's feet can extend the edge comfortably. You can make the firm surface more comfortable with a length of foam rubber.

The real challenge presented by a dining room table is its height, since this is the main source of occupational strain. There are various ways of adjusting height relative to the table, such as using blocks under the legs to raise the table, or using a broad plank or running board to raise the massager. Experience suggests that it is always advisable to adapt the environment to the table rather than take a saw to the table itself.

TOWELS

Top of the list of required equipment is a generous towel or cloth to cover the patient's body. This is a physiological necessity, even in warmer countries, since the temperature of the part of the body not being massaged is actually lowered and needs to be insulated. Also, the parts of the body that are being massaged need covering immediately after treatment, or they, too, will cool down quickly.

Toweling is a neutral form of covering, and most people associate it with the unwinding of tension. A covering also serves to preserve modesty. This is important, not from fear of sexual intimacy but because it is symbolic of the practitioner's carefulness. Towels may also be used for other practical purposes such as pillowing, or as wedges to help release tension in the joints.

OILS AND POWDER

Some patients prefer oil massage, while others find the idea of being "oiled-up" unpleasant. Good-quality vegetable oils are very useful for sports massage and with children or older adults, where the pressure of strokes needs to be deflected. Add the oil a little at a time to your hand so it is slightly warmed, rather than pouring cold oil directly onto the patient. When using essential oils, take great care not to cause irritation to the eyes, or around the eyes. These oils can also damage a patient's clothing.

Talcum powder has no therapeutic properties. It is used by trainee therapists until the effleurage stroke is perfected, and has no other use in massage.

SCREENS

Some practitioners offer their patients a screen for use when they undress. This obviously provides the patient with a sense of privacy and saves the practitioner any embarrassment; it can also make undressing and dressing easier, since the patient is not self-distracted. Undressing behavior can communicate a lot to an observant massager, however, and this possibility is denied if the patient uses a screen.

SOFT AND WARM
*Soft, fresh towels are essential equipment for massage.
They keep the patient warm and provide a welcome
sense of being cared for.*

ENVIRONMENT

The massage environment should be warm and airy, with no taint of previous treatments. Inadequate ventilation may make the patient feel drowsy when sitting up, and it is a good idea to open the windows wide after the final session. The hygiene of the couch can be maintained by changing the towels or using strips of paper sheeting from a roll. If you are giving more than one essential oil treatment during a therapy session, intersperse them with a treatment that does not use oil of any kind. Sunlight entering the treatment room is very therapeutic if it is directed on to the patient's body. Artificial lighting can be subdued, and should not confront the patient's eyes. Background music may be useful when the patient is on the couch, but check: what may sound appropriate to you may not appeal to the patient, either at the beginning of massage or once treatment is underway, and this may frustrate your efforts to achieve a relaxed atmosphere.

DRESS   CODE

CLOTHING
It is better to have your clothing arranged before massage so that you do not have to remove any garments during a treatment. A warm but lightweight top with tight or three-quarter-length sleeves allows free movement.

SHOES
Always wear shoes at the initial consultation, but, if, for comfort, you prefer bare feet when giving treatment, you can remove your shoes after massage has begun and replace them when you finish.

HAIR
If your hair hangs forward over your eyes, or might come into contact with the patient during head or face massage, tie it back. Your hair should be well-combed before treatment to reduce the chance of loose hairs falling onto the patient.

HANDS
As well as washing your hands – using a nailbrush – before treatments, remove all large rings, watches and bracelets. Your nails should be short and unpainted. Use hand-energizing exercises to prepare them for giving strokes, and if necessary soften the palms with a simple hand cream.

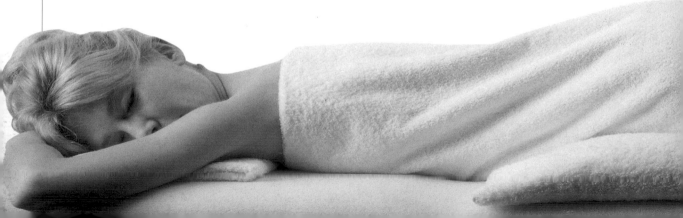

SELF-HELP

Professional massagers practice a form of "cool-down" at the end of each treatment session, which helps detach them from their patients' physical and emotional problems. Everyone has their own technique, which may involve stretching movements of the hands, rotating the trunk, traction self-treatments, and meditation. As you gain practice you will devise a self-help routine to suit your own needs.

BASIC PRECAUTIONS

There are occasions when applied massage has to be suitably modified or, rarely, restricted to minimal treatment. Massage practitioners are guided in this by the patient's medical history at the initial consultation. At the same time, the practitioner records any personal reservations or reluctance the patient may have toward a particular aspect of treatment.

Since some patients may not feel obliged to be perfectly candid about their case history, professional massage practitioners often ask their patients to sign a disclaimer that acknowledges a shared responsibility for the outcome of any course of treatment.

Some patients seek complementary therapies to fill the gap left by discontinued conventional care. In such cases it is essential to be alert to any known pathological processes or psychological conditions that might make the patient's response to massage less predictable. If there is any doubt, a massage therapist can usually consult with the patient's medical practitioner to discuss suitable treatment.

PADS AND WEDGES
Folded towels and pillows can be used to provide padding beneath sensitive areas of the body, and as wedges to help disperse tension in the joints.

"WATCH POINTS"

Massage is a sensitive and considerate therapy. Whole-body treatment may be modified or withheld if the patient:

- HAS A DEGENERATIVE/INFLAMMATORY DISEASE
- IS UNDERGOING MANIPULATIVE THERAPY, such as osteopathy
- IS ON MAJOR MEDICATION, such as steroids
- HAS RECENTLY HAD SURGERY
- HAS RECENTLY BEEN INJURED (within 48 hours)
- IS PREGNANT OR MENSTRUATING (when she can be shown self-massage techniques)

GENERAL RULES

There are times when whole-body massage may be contraindicated. These include during pregnancy, in the period immediately after injury, and during the acute stages of any disease. Chronic conditions, if degenerative, should also be given only modified massage. As a general rule, avoid giving pressure or percussion strokes to areas of inflammation. Slow, deep pressure strokes can be given to adjacent areas to bring relief, but otherwise the patient's preference is a reliable guide.

These points apply equally to aromatherapy. Furthermore, the use of essential oils should be discontinued both when pregnancy has been established, and during the early stages of breast-feeding. At low dosage (one percent or less), essential oils may be introduced gradually from one month after the birth. The primary contraindication in aromatherapy is simple: the patient does not like the scent of the treatment oil offered. The commonly ascribed actions of essential oils are not reliable and should not overrule the patient's preference.

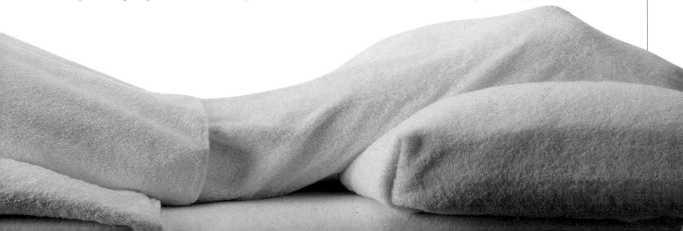

GIVING A MASSAGE

Most adults approach their first massage with a variety of preconceptions. Regardless of your approach, your partner may expect massage to be an athletic or hedonistic experience, be both threatening and relaxing, daringly sexual, or completely clinical. The actual massage will soon clarify these ideas, for what is really at issue for your partner is how he or she reacts to being handled. This in turn depends on your partner's experience of physical contact throughout life, from early childhood. Giving a massage involves a lot more than simply applying the strokes.

MOST PATIENTS ARE particularly vulnerable to the first and last touch of massage. You must make sure that the beginning and ending of your treatments are slow and gentle, careful and reassuring. The sequence of massage can also be relevant, since starting on a vulnerable part of the body can create resistance. Hand massage (see page 104) can be a good way to begin as it provides a familiar point of contact, and you can talk to each other in the usual way.

CLEARING THE AIR
The preconceptions that people bring to massage can affect the way they approach their first experience of therapy. Clearing up such preconceptions is an important first step in any course of treatment.

As you proceed, try to maintain a relaxed, confident attitude and a flexible treatment plan. It is essential that your patients sense your sincerity, enjoy the atmosphere of the treatment environment, and appreciate your expertise, but you should not feel you have to make an effort in presentation. Patients are subtly affected by tension in the massager, so it is best to avoid intense concentration and let your mind freewheel a little.

What actually occurs in a treatment is the responsibility of both people. During a massage, either person can sense when something does not feel right; if this happens, stop. Good massage depends on communication, so if your wires are crossed it may be better to postpone the treatment to another day.

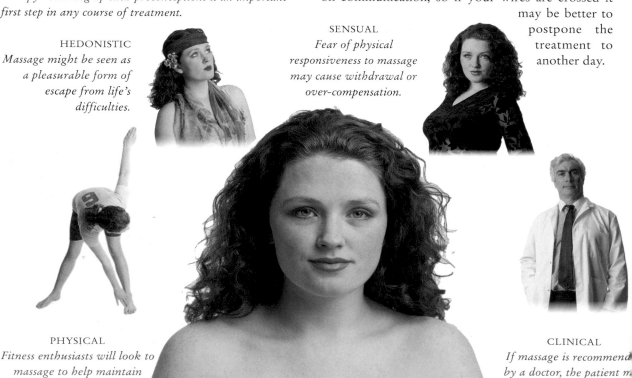

HEDONISTIC
Massage might be seen as a pleasurable form of escape from life's difficulties.

SENSUAL
Fear of physical responsiveness to massage may cause withdrawal or over-compensation.

PHYSICAL
Fitness enthusiasts will look to massage to help maintain muscle tone.

CLINICAL
If massage is recommend by a doctor, the patient m expect that the treatment be a clinical experience.

TENSION REMEDY

The habit of raising the shoulders in response to anxiety is understandable. It is likely, however, that the shoulder of the preferred hand will get "hitched up" and remain tense even after the initial cause of tension has subsided. The treatment which follows is very simple to give and can, in fact, be done as a self-treatment. The practitioner gives guided movements rather than strokes, and persuades the shoulder to release its tension much more effectively than the popular self-applied "shoulder-shrugging" action.

1 Stand back from your seated patient to see any discrepancies in shoulder height. The joint may appear higher, the shoulder may rotate backward, or the neck may appear shorter on the affected side.

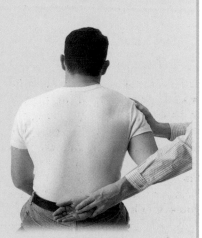

2 Place both the patient's hands in his lap. Gently lift the arm on the tenser side and fold it behind his back, within the limits of comfort.

3 Do repeated one-way effleurage from the neck to the elbow. Occasionally stroke down the front of the arm.

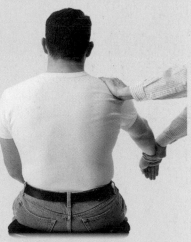

4 Support the weight of the arm and lift it up and around to the front of the body. Place one hand against the collar bone and use the other to extend the arm forward. Hold for a few seconds, then replace the hand into the patient's lap.

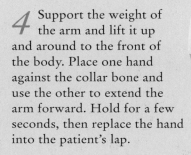

5 The shoulder that was tighter will now be lower than the other. Apply the same treatment to the second shoulder, then repeat again only to the first. Both shoulders will now be lower.

Working Posture

FOR BEGINNERS, massage is all about learning how to use their hands, but with experience they soon appreciate how much the whole body is involved. This means that if the posture of the massager is not correct, giving massage can become a very strenuous experience indeed. Too much concentration on the strokes can lead to tension in the forearms. Constantly leaning over the treatment couch can be hazardous for the lower back. Massaging also tends to round the shoulders and restrict breathing.

SOME TREATMENTS ARE more physically demanding than others, but it is important to develop an efficient technique that will protect you, the massager, from occupational strain. Since giving massage provides an opportunity to be physically active, however, there are also physical benefits to be enjoyed. Indeed, most practitioners welcome a list of appointments, for a single treatment tends to leave them feeling just warmed up and ready for more.

THE BACK

Any massage practitioner worthy of the name would normally advise against working in a position that involves continually leaning over. If you are to remain free of back problems you must take special safeguards and develop a faultless technique. The poise of your back muscles allows you the uninterrupted use of your hands that you need to provide the detailed manipulations of massage. It is your legs, however, that give rhythm and weight to the depth of treatment, and confusion between these two areas is potentially damaging to the lower back.

Fortunately, accurate application of effleurage, the most commonly performed massage stroke, is very connecting for the massager's body. It allows the muscles to stretch and realign themselves without disturbing the continuity of the massage treatment. Generous use of effleurage, therefore, has advantages for both patient and practitioner.

This is especially relevant if the treatment has to be given from the kneeling position, which greatly reduces flexibility. If you are unable to use a table, and kneeling massage is the only option, you can obtain a specially designed low massage stool that fits across the feet. Giving massage from a seated position also reduces flexibility, however, and this method should only be considered for short treatments.

KNEELING
Try to avoid giving massage from a kneeling position, because the fixed leg posture you have to adopt will build up strain in your back.

STAMINA AND POSTURE

Some people doubt whether they will have the stamina required to give effective massage. Others feel that postural problems of their own may be a hindrance to treating others. In fact, the opposite can be true. Giving good massage promotes fitness in the giver, and there are numerous examples where massaging has helped people understand and remedy their own back problems. When performed properly, massage movements are flowing and economical, and encourage strength and flexibility in the massager. Aches and pains are often the result of overexertion and nervousness in our posture generally, which learning massage can help reduce. Despite this, there are key areas of potential strain for massagers, and it is useful to be aware of these. If you are giving regular massage you should use self-treatment techniques such as traction and low back pain relief (see page 194), and be sure to benefit from regular massage yourself.

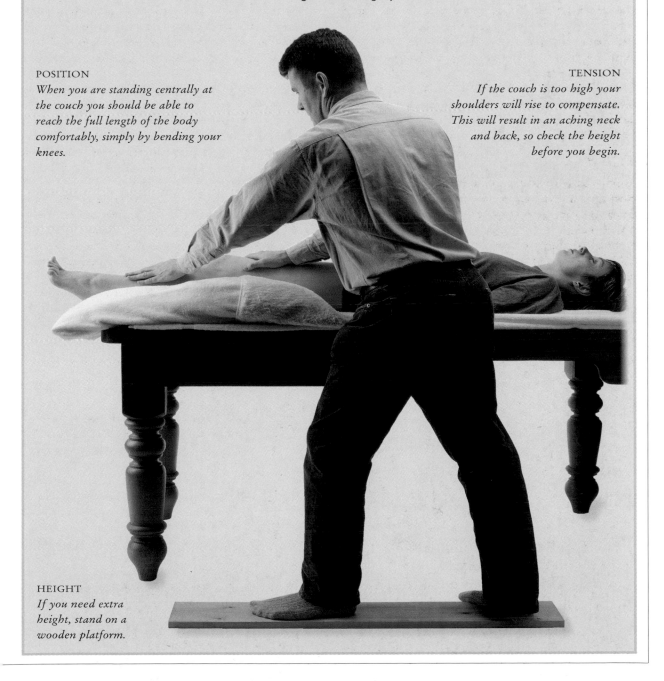

POSITION
When you are standing centrally at the couch you should be able to reach the full length of the body comfortably, simply by bending your knees.

TENSION
If the couch is too high your shoulders will rise to compensate. This will result in an aching neck and back, so check the height before you begin.

HEIGHT
If you need extra height, stand on a wooden platform.

Your Hands

THE HANDS, with their unique combination of muscular dexterity and nervous sensitivity, have been described as "the visible portion of the brain." Free from locomotive responsibility, they have developed into powerful precision tools in which the thumbs, used in opposition with the fingers, are capable of tasks requiring both strength and delicacy. The sensitivity of the hands is vital in massage, since it provides direct communication with the unspoken thoughts and feelings which are expressed in the tension of the patient's body.

EACH OF YOUR hands is a supremely flexible construction, containing eight wrist bones, five palm bones and 14 finger bones. It is moved by tiny muscles within the hand and by larger, powerful muscles operating by remote control from the forearm. This arrangement means that, despite the constant activity of your hands, they never enlarge from exercise but retain their slender, delicate shape.

The refinement of coordination in the human hand is such that it is the earliest expression of physical control by the infant. Even newborn babies can exert a vice-like grip, so that young children can be relied upon to grasp precious objects safely. Relatively difficult tasks requiring manual skill are learned a little later, but they are often learned quickly. Soon a variety of functioning is developed from the basic power and precision grips to give the dexterity that makes massage possible.

The admirable delicacy of your hands is not only an esthetic quality. The thousands of sensory nerve endings transmit the most subtle information back from the environment to your body's central nervous system for processing. Your hands can distinguish between pleasurable and threatening sensations. They are capable of identifying size and shape, texture and temperature. Your hands are also faithful recorders which remember sensations. This is why the second massage treatment is usually more influential, since your hands recognize the patient and go quickly towards the sources of discomfort in the muscles.

The expressiveness – or lack of it – in the hands can mirror inner conditions. Being therapeutic tools, it is not surprising that a therapist's hands are regarded as highly emotional structures, as the expression "laying on hands" suggests. The patient's hands are, of course, also emotional, and can make equally symbolic gestures. Hands can adopt mini-postures, such as empty clenched fists. They can drop things, become suddenly very moist, and are subject to nail-biting mutilation. All these actions can speak louder than words to a sensitive observer.

SENSITIVE HANDS

The brain and the spinal cord form the central processing unit of the nervous system, receiving messages from the body and sending instructions back. The relative sensitivity of the different parts of the body can be seen from the size of the relevant section of the diagram shown here. The face, lips and tongue are well-supplied with sensory nerves, while the trunk and the limbs are much less sensitive, The fingers and the palms of the hands are also extremely sensitive, allowing the massager direct access to the emotional and physical state of the patient as expressed through the tension of their body.

Trunk — Neck — Arm — Palm — Legs — Foot — Toes — Fourth finger — Third finger — Second finger — First finger — Thumb — Eyes — Face — Lips — Tongue and throat

AWARENESS GAME

Massage practitioners learn to rely on the information received through their hands in developing appropriate treatments. While the skin over the palms is relatively thick on its surface, the fingertips contain a massive number of sensory nerve endings, second only to the soles of the feet for heightened sensitivity. This exercise illustrates how dependable our sense of touch can be in recording information. At first, try the game on the palms, then make it a little harder by using the slightly less sensitive skin of the lower arm. Eventually, try it on the back, where the nerves are more spaced out and recording detailed sensation is far more challenging.

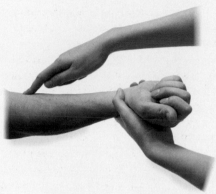

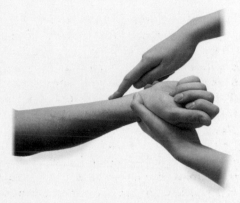

1 Sit alongside a partner so that he can easily turn away to avoid seeing you. Touch his bared forearm. Make a simple impression, say a diagonal line with your fingertip, from elbow to wrist. The partner should then reproduce this from memory on your forearm.

2 If the reconstruction is accurate, repeat the first movement and then add a further impression, such as three or four "dots." Ask your partner to reproduce the initial and extended stimulation.

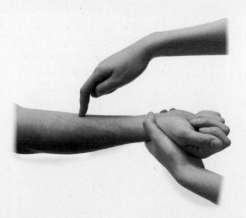

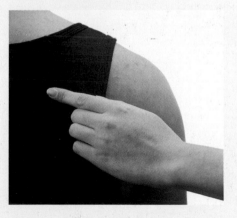

3 Continue with another type of contact, such as a wavy line. If the partner is successful in reproducing the whole sequence, continue to add more and varied sensations until they are impossible to reconstruct. Then swap roles and start over again.

4 Try the exercise over the shoulder blade. This is not a particularly sensitive area, but it is a site of common tension and therefore a useful place to increase awareness of the slightest pressure.

WARMING UP FOR MASSAGE

WE BRING BUSY and sometimes tired hands to massage. Our motor skills are focused in them from the moment we awaken each day, yet our hands are situated almost as far as they could be from the sources of fresh circulation and nervous energy. Like our feet, they have no muscles within them to help dispel tiredness, and the muscles that do control them often suffer from repetitive strain. So to make sure that massage does not place further demands on your hands, practice the following exercises both before and after giving treatments.

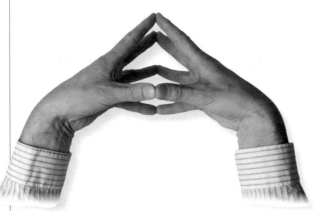

2 Reunite your hands and press them firmly together. Keep pressing and lower them until they are in line with your elbows. Maintain a steady stretching pressure for about 10 seconds, with no bouncing. To increase the effect, rotate your forearms so your fingertips touch your body and then point away again, and release slowly. Repeat 6–10 times.

1 Place your hands together in front of your chest. Press the tips of your fingers together so as to separate the rest of your hands and widen the space between each set of fingers. Make 10 gentle bounces of the straight fingers to extend the stretch into the palms of your hands.

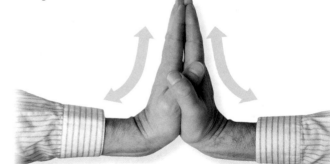

3 Make soft fists, with your thumbs tucked in beneath your fingers. Hold for five seconds. Squeeze equally with all the fingers and hold for a further five seconds.

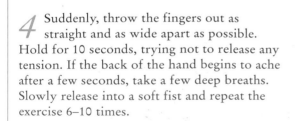

4 Suddenly, throw the fingers out as straight and as wide apart as possible. Hold for 10 seconds, trying not to release any tension. If the back of the hand begins to ache after a few seconds, take a few deep breaths. Slowly release into a soft fist and repeat the exercise 6–10 times.

TOUCHING AND LISTENING

Some people recommend giving massage in silence, presumably because they feel that spoken conversation interferes with the subtler interactions of treatment. In practice, however, it is a good idea to preface the deeper movements of massage with a few introductory remarks about their intended effects. Some patients may also need reassurance about the unexpected reactions that can occur in early appointments.

SOMETIMES THE PATIENT may have something to say. Massage is often resorted to because it represents a form of communication that is not available in day-to-day life. And while massage aims to facilitate physical expression, it is not unusual for a patient experiencing the benefit of treatment to feel a need to speak about his or her problems in life. Most practitioners welcome this response, because it suggests that they are beginning to share a trusting relationship. Others do not appreciate this aspect of massage practice, however, and there are some who, embarrassed by their lack of formal listening skills, indirectly discourage it.

In practice, it is not necessary to either discourage or encourage personal disclosure, provided the principles of massage are adhered to. By using massage therapy as a listening process in itself, you need not feel under pressure to understand what the patient is saying.

During massage your hands are in somatic conversation with your patient's muscles, whose tensions often contain feelings of need that are too urgent to be openly and directly verbalized. When they are, you can assume that, having chosen to receive massage, the patient expects to receive more massage rather than verbal counseling. The strokes of massage are designed to be gently provocative in countering tensions, and confidently communicating with the feelings behind words.

TALKING HANDS
Massage is about communication through touch, but this should not discourage verbal communication. If the patient feels the need to say something, let him go ahead, but try not to get involved in earnest discussion. Reply with your hands, rather than your voice.

HAND MASSAGE

MASSAGE OF THE hand makes a good beginning to a treatment. It allows eye contact between the participants and permits easy conversation about how the massage is progressing. For a new patient the hand provides a very useful introduction to massage, and meanwhile the practitioner finds it a valuable guide to the condition of the rest of the patient's body. The tension of the hand, in its tiny muscles, in the ease of its joints, and the warmth of its circulation, gives an indication of general tension in the system. Apart from its relaxing local benefits, massage of the hands reduces pressure at the neck by nervous reflex.

1 Ask the patient to lie down and rest her right arm on a small pillow, with the elbow flexed. Contain her hand between your own for a few moments.

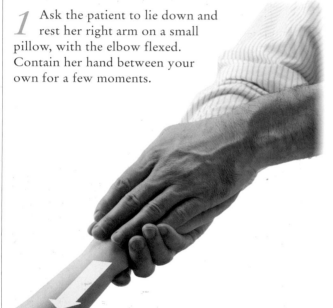

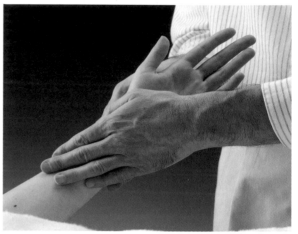

2 Give effleurage by sliding both hands steadily from the fingertip to the forearm. Apply only very light pressure.

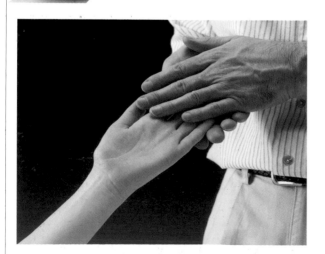

3 Give return effleurage with equally light pressure, back to the fingertips. Repeat the effleurage six times.

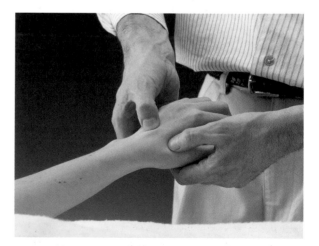

4 Turn the palm over and begin petrissage. Using your thumbs, squeeze all over the back of the hand, both on the bones and in the spaces between, for 30 seconds.

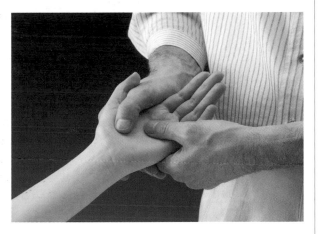

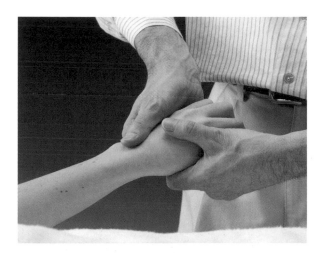

5 Effleurage the hand using spreading thumb pressures, diverging to the left and right, from the knuckles down to the wrists.

6 Turn the hand over and petrissage the palm for 30 seconds. For this stage your thumbs should be placed flatter than in step 4. Give special attention to the patient's own thumb.

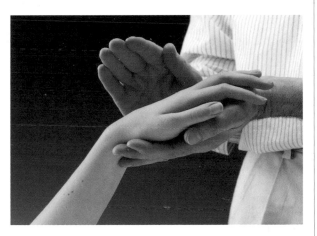

8 Support the patient's hand and, using all your fingers, give light, sharp tapping to front and back for 20 seconds.

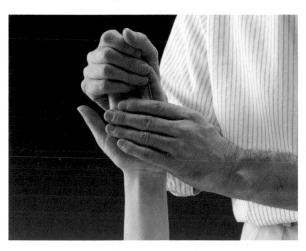

7 Holding the fingers to bring the forearm upright, do firm effleurage through the hand, six times to the front and six times to the back.

9 Give fingertip effleurage from the fingers down into the forearm, with the strokes becoming progressively lighter and slower, for 30 seconds. Complete the massage by containing the hand softly, as in step 1. Place the hand across the abdomen, but, before treating the other hand, ask the patient to compare the feeling in each. The positive difference will demonstrate the beneficial effects of massage.

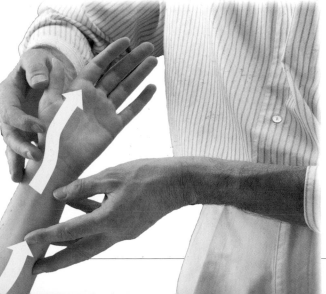

THERAPEUTIC WHOLE-BODY MASSAGE

THE CONVENTION OF beginning a massage with a back treatment is open to negotiation between patient and practitioner, but inexperienced massagers may prefer to be confronted by the relatively impersonal aspect of the back since this helps focus their concentration. This sequence is designed to bring about a sense of concentration shared between practitioner and patient. It helps create a calm atmosphere that is settling for the patient, and meanwhile the massager gets the opportunity to practice body awareness before introducing the strokes.

1 Have your partner lie face down, and cover her with towels to keep her warm and relaxed.

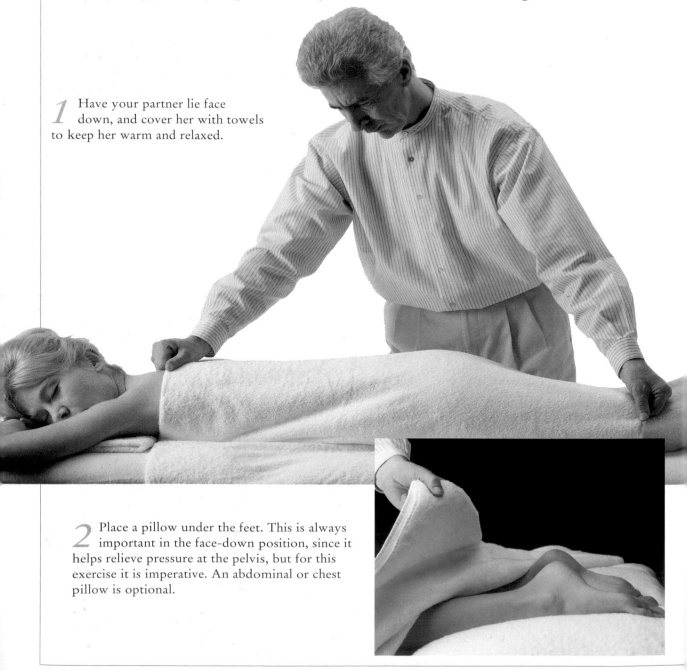

2 Place a pillow under the feet. This is always important in the face-down position, since it helps relieve pressure at the pelvis, but for this exercise it is imperative. An abdominal or chest pillow is optional.

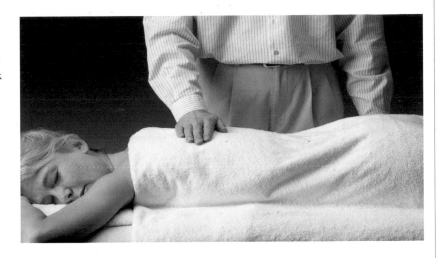

3 Place one hand lightly on the middle of your partner's back and the other over her pelvis. Invite her to breathe deeply and slowly. An obvious movement shows the chest rising and falling with each breath.

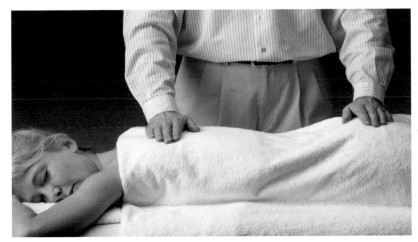

4 Focus your other hand on the back of your partner's pelvis. Be aware of any movement corresponding to the breathing movement of the chest. Observe a few more breaths.

5 Now place your other hand lightly on the back of your partner's head. Be aware of any "breathing" at the head. Transfer your attention back to the hand on the pelvis. It may be more obvious now that the pelvis does indeed have a breathing rhythm.

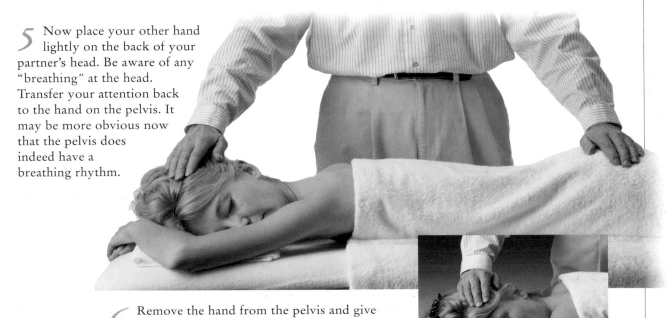

6 Remove the hand from the pelvis and give complete attention to the head. The movement here is very subtle, resembling a vibration. A few moments' concentration here will establish a conducive atmosphere for further treatment.

BACK MASSAGE

M ASSAGE OF THE back has become an established way to begin a whole-body treatment. The major muscles of posture are situated to the back of the body, and since the spinal nerve roots are accessible from the back, it might be a logical place to begin. However, back massage can be physically challenging to perform. A very tense patient is an unyielding surface to warm up on, and the shape and size of some patients may force the massager into a lot of bending and reaching. These problems can be overcome by liberal use of effleurage, which ensures that back massage provides a relaxing start for both giver and receiver.

1 Stand to the right of the patient. Fold the upper towel back from the neck to the highest point of the lower back at the sacrum. Secure it by tucking a little under each side of the pelvis.

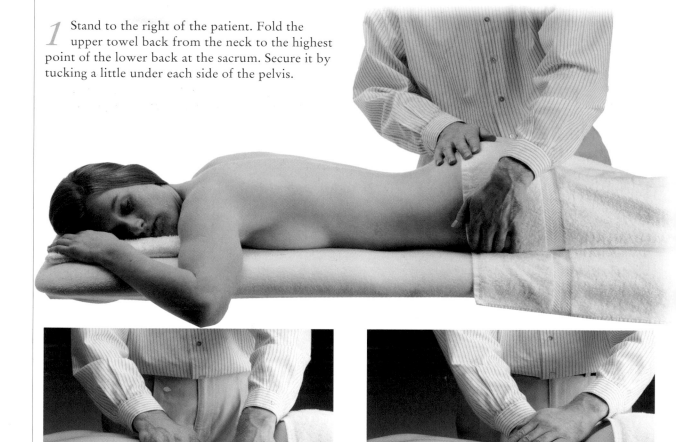

2 Effleurage the back with a smooth rhythm for two minutes. Relax your fingers and thumbs for maximum palm contact and follow the contours of the body. Keep your shoulders loose and bend your knees to reach up, down, and across the body.

3 Focus on the patient's lower back. Make a "reinforced hand" by placing your left hand passively upon your right. Gradually increase the depth of effleurage, making sweeping circles between chest and pelvis.

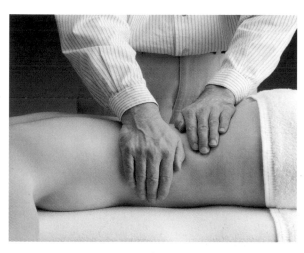

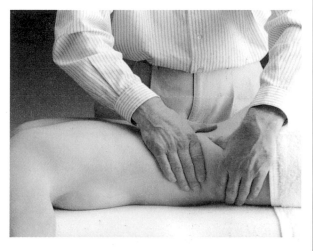

4 Reach over to the far side of the body and give firm effleurage for 10 seconds, from the edge of the waist toward the spine.

5 Knead the waist on that side for 30 seconds, overlapping a little on the side of the chest and using more pressure over the rim of the pelvis.

6 Give 10 slow, deep effleurage strokes toward the spine, and then repeat all the movements for the waist. During the second series of kneading strokes you can usually apply deeper pressure.

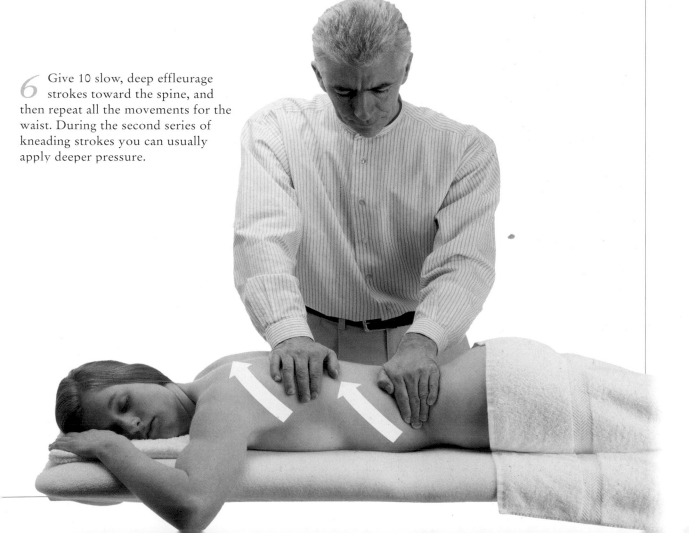

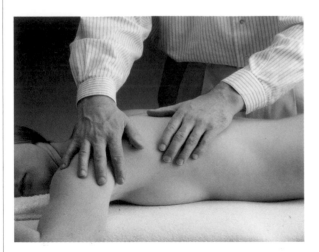

7 Do light, continuous effleurage, progressively moving from the waist to the side of the chest, upper back, and shoulder.

8 Petrissage the edge of the chest, from the lower ribs to the underarm and back again, six times. If your partner finds this stimulates a tickle, draw her elbow a little nearer her chest and begin again.

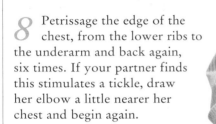

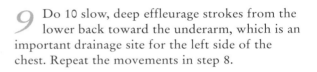

9 Do 10 slow, deep effleurage strokes from the lower back toward the underarm, which is an important drainage site for the left side of the chest. Repeat the movements in step 8.

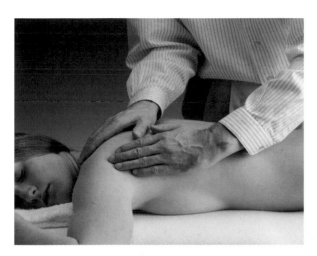

10 Continue via smooth effleurage to the top of the shoulder. At this stage it is important to check that your patient's head position allows free access to her shoulder. If necessary, ask her to gently turn her head away from the massage strokes.

11 Using your left hand, petrissage with strong thumb strokes along the top edge of the shoulder, holding gently with the fingertips. This is a universally popular massage stroke.

12 Using your fingertips to balance, give firm thumb pressure from the base of the neck to the base of the rib-cage on either side of the spine. Press up and down six times.

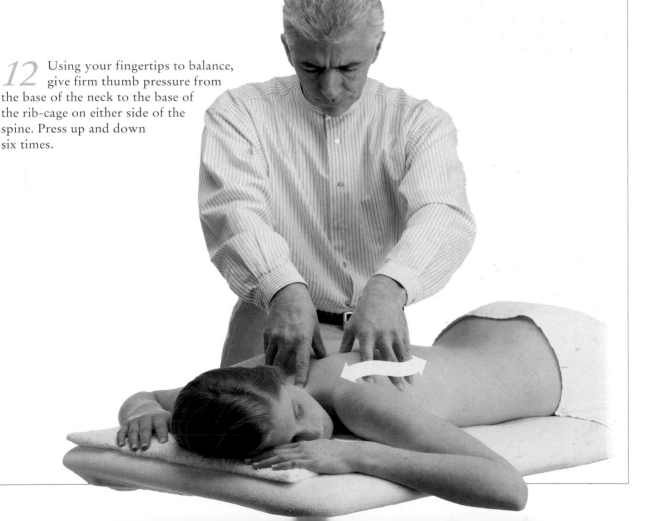

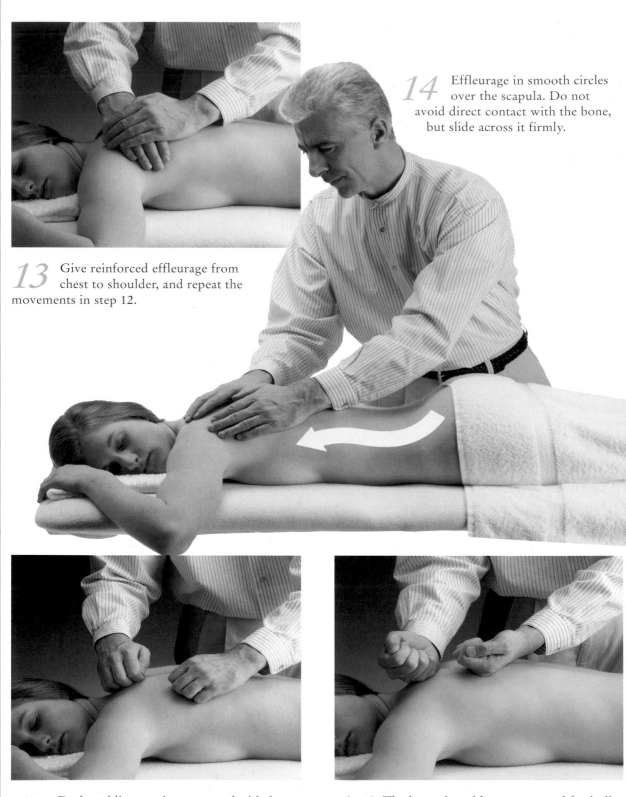

14 Effleurage in smooth circles over the scapula. Do not avoid direct contact with the bone, but slide across it firmly.

13 Give reinforced effleurage from chest to shoulder, and repeat the movements in step 12.

15 Do knuckling petrissage over the blade, around the edges, near the spine, and toward the shoulder joint, for 30 seconds. Use the smaller knuckles on the slender shoulder and the middle knuckles where there is more muscle.

16 The larger knuckles are reserved for bulky shoulders. Draw your upturned hand roughly over the scapula and toward the spine.

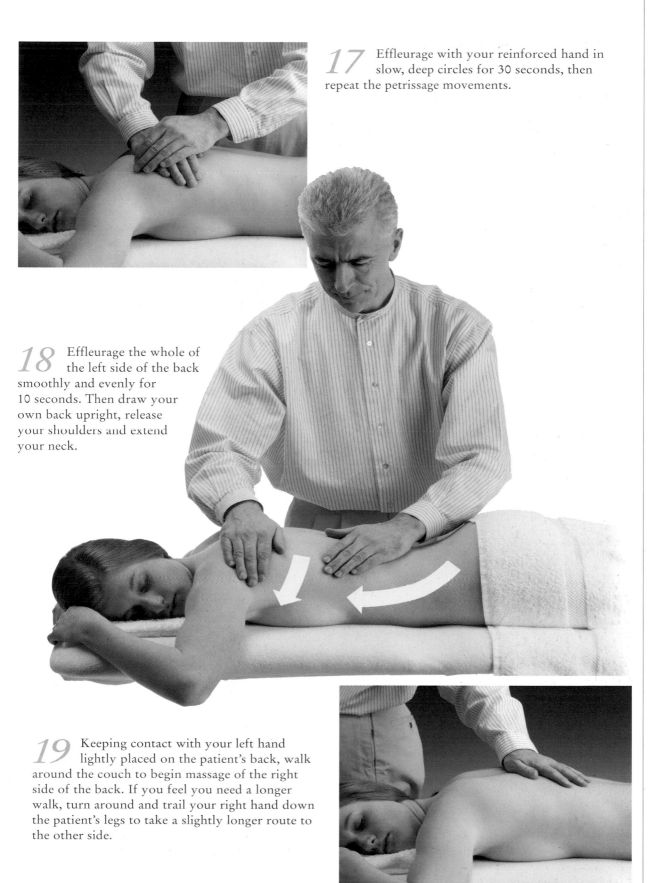

17 Effleurage with your reinforced hand in slow, deep circles for 30 seconds, then repeat the petrissage movements.

18 Effleurage the whole of the left side of the back smoothly and evenly for 10 seconds. Then draw your own back upright, release your shoulders and extend your neck.

19 Keeping contact with your left hand lightly placed on the patient's back, walk around the couch to begin massage of the right side of the back. If you feel you need a longer walk, turn around and trail your right hand down the patient's legs to take a slightly longer route to the other side.

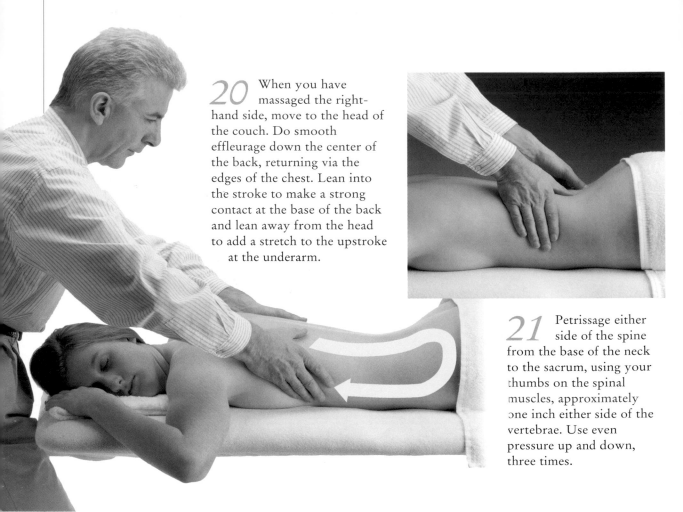

20 When you have massaged the right-hand side, move to the head of the couch. Do smooth effleurage down the center of the back, returning via the edges of the chest. Lean into the stroke to make a strong contact at the base of the back and lean away from the head to add a stretch to the upstroke at the underarm.

21 Petrissage either side of the spine from the base of the neck to the sacrum, using your thumbs on the spinal muscles, approximately one inch either side of the vertebrae. Use even pressure up and down, three times.

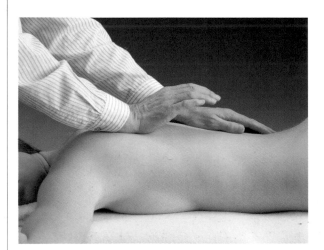

22 Alternatively, and for strong backs, use the heels of your hands. Give a firm push on the sacrum to complete the downstroke and a lighter squeeze between the scapulas on return. If you are unable to reach the whole length of the back, stand at the corner of the couch in a three-quarters position.

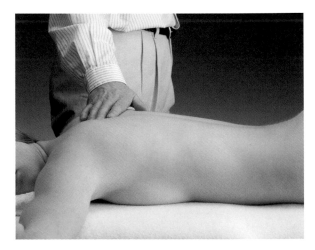

23 Return to the right-hand side of the couch, taking a short or long walk and maintaining contact on the back or leg as before.

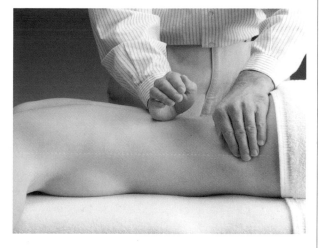

24 Percuss the whole back for 30 seconds, using hacking. Keep your hands close to the skin and begin slowly, building speed gradually. Give special attention to the tops of the shoulders and the edge of the chest.

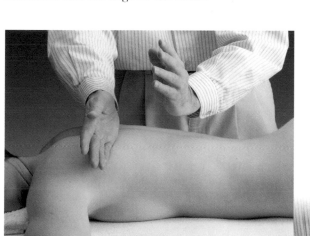

25 The lower back and rim of the pelvis may now be cupped for 20 seconds. Start slowly as before, if necessary keeping the heel of your hand resting on the body to maintain the cupped position.

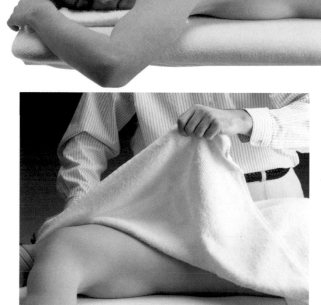

26 Repeat the effleurage with which you began the massage. Effleurage for one minute, making the strokes lighter and slower, with less palm and more fingertip contact, until you are barely touching the body. Let your hands come to rest lightly on the lower and upper back.

27 Pause for a few seconds, then cover the back by carefully drawing up the towel to the back of the patient's head and securing it around her shoulders.

LEG MASSAGE

SUPPORTING THE WHOLE weight of the body, capable of both exquisite poise and powerful locomotion, the leg muscles are very effective self-massagers. Their movements overcome the strong gravitational resistance to blood flow in the veins, and in this way they contribute toward an efficient circulation. In the past, patients with cardiovascular disorders were ordered to bed and told not to move, but today they are advised to make active leg movements to relieve strain on the heart. Symptoms of cramp and varicosity in the legs indicate tiredness, so a massage treatment is an opportunity to give the legs a well-deserved treat.

1 Uncover the leg from toes to buttock. Tuck the top of the towel in at the waist and wrap it around the other leg. Effleurage the leg continuously for 30 seconds from the heel to the buttock, looping around to return.

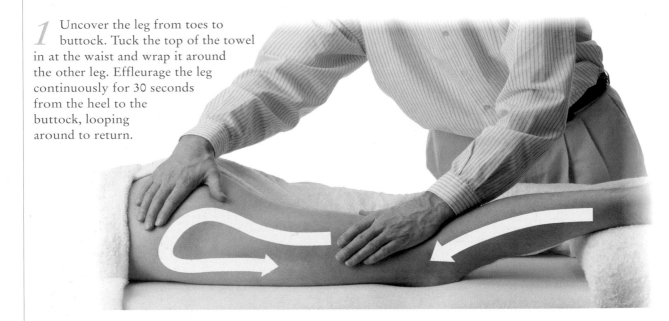

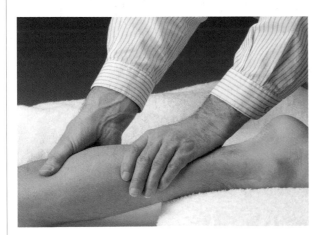

2 By alternating your hands, apply rolling, diverging effleurage on the lower leg from the heel to the back of the knee, six times.

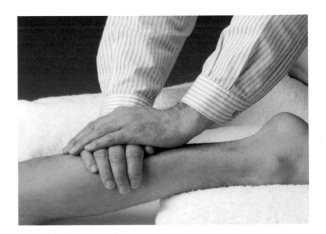

3 Using the reinforced hand technique, apply deep effleurage to the lower leg six times. Then repeat the movements in step 2.

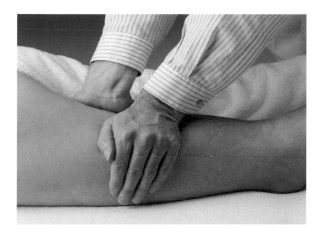

4 Give light effleurage to the back of the thigh. Place the heel of your hands to either side of the knee and gently press up the hamstring muscles, converging on the fold of the buttock.

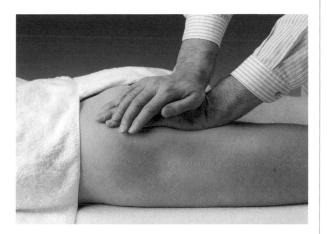

5 Press the heel of your lower hand firmly on the middle of the upper thigh. Effleurage the thigh from the back of the knee, with reinforced hand, six times. Repeat the movements in step 4.

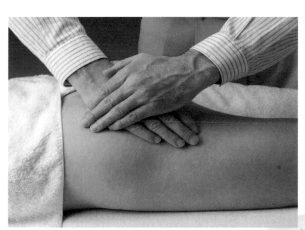

6 Do circular, counterclockwise effleurage of the buttock with your reinforced hand for 10 seconds, sweeping your hands around to include the outside of the thigh.

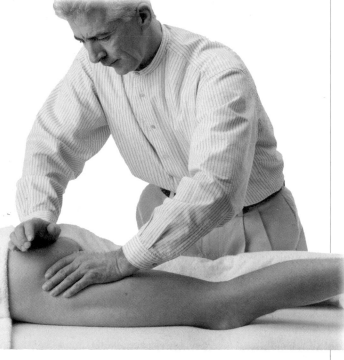

7 Knead the buttock muscles, keeping close palm contact to avoid pinching, or use the heel of your hand to roll over the muscles. Continue for 30 seconds. Effleurage deeply and repeat six times.

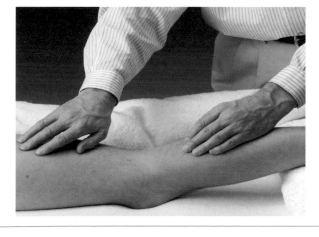

8 Effleurage the whole leg with a deeper upstroke six times, then effleurage montonously, lighter, slower, and with decreasing contact until you are using only your fingertips. Cover the leg, wrapping the towel all around, then massage the other leg.

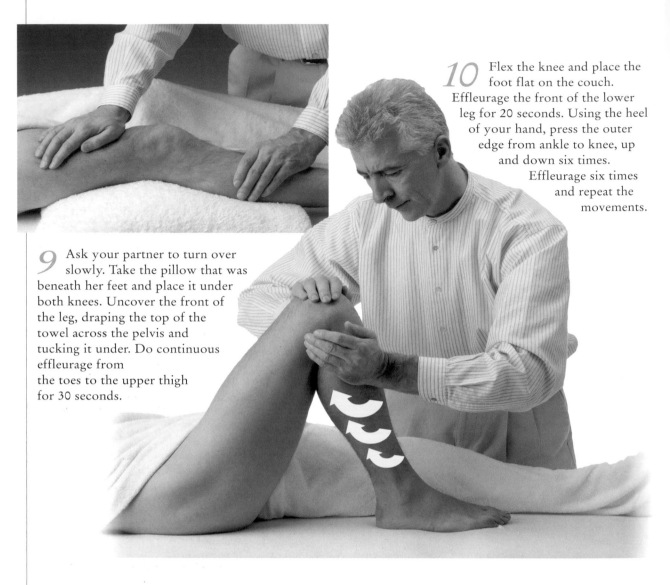

10 Flex the knee and place the foot flat on the couch. Effleurage the front of the lower leg for 20 seconds. Using the heel of your hand, press the outer edge from ankle to knee, up and down six times. Effleurage six times and repeat the movements.

9 Ask your partner to turn over slowly. Take the pillow that was beneath her feet and place it under both knees. Uncover the front of the leg, draping the top of the towel across the pelvis and tucking it under. Do continuous effleurage from the toes to the upper thigh for 30 seconds.

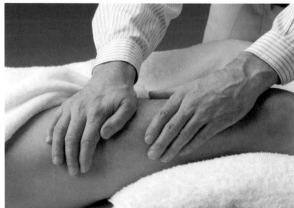

11 Extend the patient's leg carefully, then effleurage the whole of the upper leg for 20 seconds.

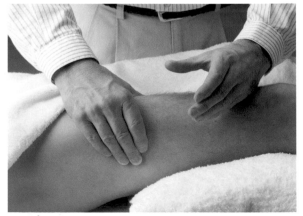

12 Place your outstretched hands across the front of the thigh and knead up and down six times. Use double-handed strokes on well-developed muscles. Effleurage six times and repeat the movements.

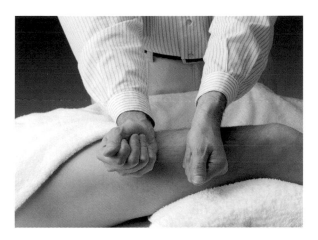

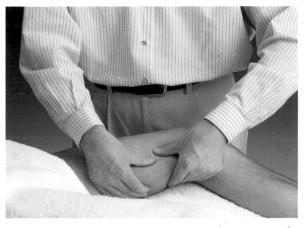

13 Do pummeling on the outer thigh, up and down, six times. Keep your hands very close to the leg to avoid percussing. Effleurage six times and repeat the movements. Then effleurage lightly before the next stroke.

14 Petrissage the inner leg by placing your fingertips well underneath the leg at the knee. Work along the thigh, lightening the stroke until you are squeezing only softly at the two-thirds point. Go up and down six times. Effleurage six times and repeat. Make the final effleurage from the inside of the knee to the outside of the pelvis.

15 Stand at waist level, facing toward the feet. Lean forward and effleurage by firmly drawing your hands along the leg as you lean back, bending your knees. Lift your hands briefly to return to the foot and repeat six times. Cover and massage the other leg.

PRECAUTION

Varicose veins Avoid direct pressure but give light effleurage.
Low back pain The buttocks contain nerves that are affected by pressure in the lower back, so kneading may increase tension. If so, do slow, deep squeezing, holding for a few seconds.
Lymph nodes Do not apply pressure directly behind the knee or beyond two thirds of the inner thigh. These areas contain drainage points that might become irritated.

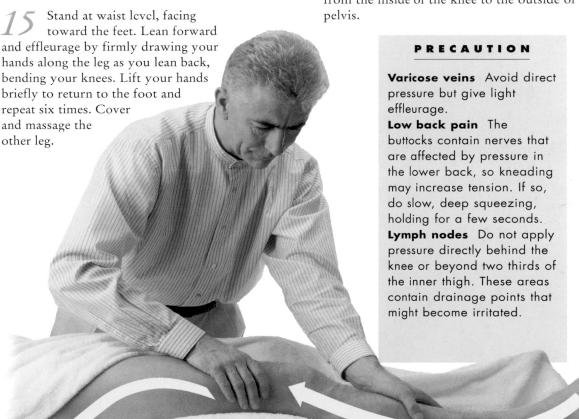

ARM MASSAGE

THE NERVES OF the body are distributed in such a way that some of those controlling the internal organs are directly related to those of the skin. This is particularly true of the chest organs and the skin on the arms, and this phenomenon enables the relaxing benefits of arm massage to be transferred to the chest interior in what is known as a reflex action. As a result, arm massage is in itself very soothing, especially for those unable to accept full body massage.

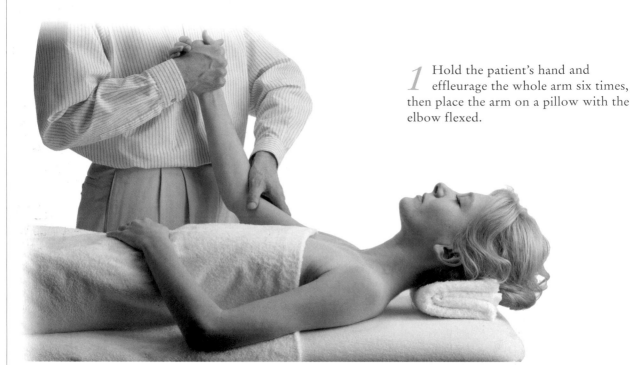

1 Hold the patient's hand and effleurage the whole arm six times, then place the arm on a pillow with the elbow flexed.

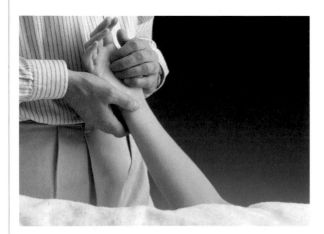

2 Rest the patient's hand against your abdomen. Effleurage the forearm by stroking from the wrist to the elbow six times, encircling the arm with alternate hands.

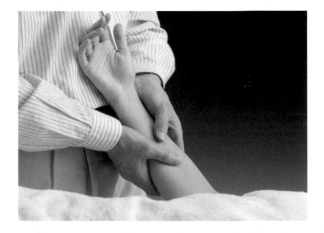

3 Petrissage softly, squeezing up and down the forearm for 20 seconds. You are massaging the muscles which move the fingers, so you may notice a response in the hand.

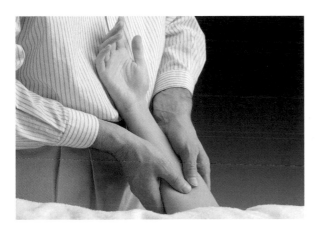

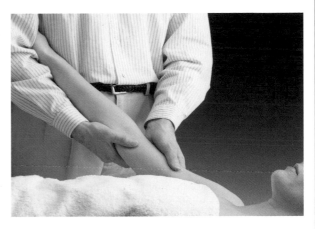

4 Effleurage deeply from wrist to elbow six times. Steady the forearm and lead with your thumbs, down the centre and to each side.

5 Extend the arm and secure it by placing it between your upper arm and chest. Effleurage from elbow to shoulder, six times.

6 Knead with both hands alternating, to the back and front of the arm, up and down for 20 seconds. Effleurage six times.

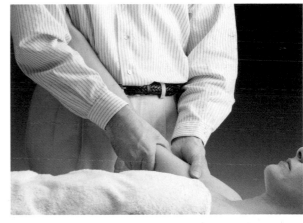

7 Raise the wrist directly above the shoulder. Apply hacking percussion to the upper arm. Complete the arm massage by firm draining, effleuraging from wrist to shoulder six times.

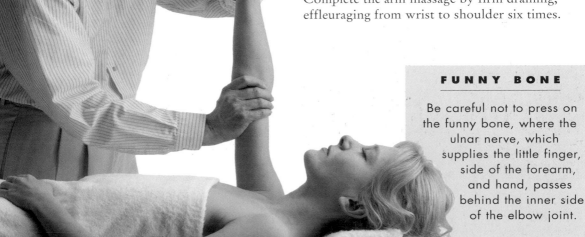

FUNNY BONE

Be careful not to press on the funny bone, where the ulnar nerve, which supplies the little finger, side of the forearm, and hand, passes behind the inner side of the elbow joint.

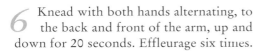

ABDOMEN MASSAGE

M OST PEOPLE ARE unsure about being touched on the abdomen. Such reserve stems from association with the pain of menstruation or acute indigestion. This should be overcome, since massage can be very helpful in both instances. There is also a possibility that abdominal massage will be resisted because it may tickle. Tickling is an odd phenomenon involving a compound of laughter and aggression, and prolonged tickling tends to eliminate the laughter. So if an abdominal stroke – or any other treatment – is considered tickly, it is best to revert to effleurage.

1 Stand close to the table at waist level and effleurage the abdomen in a clockwise circling motion, 10 times.

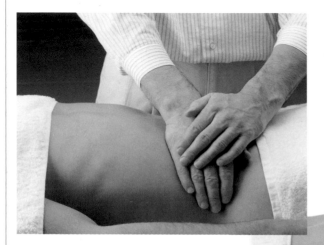

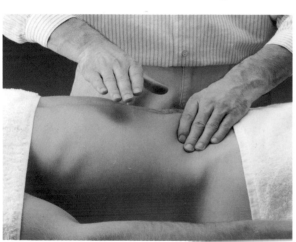

2 Do crossover pressing to relax the waist muscles. Cross your arms and place your palms against and slightly underneath the waist. Squeeze and lift, then let the body slip between your hands as you pass across the abdomen. Repeat six times, reversing your arms. Avoid pressing down on the return stroke.

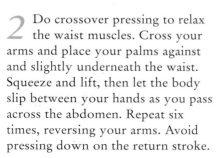

3 Petrissage the center of the abdomen using your fingertips and widely stretched thumb. Go up and down from the ribs to the front of the pelvis six times. Press lightly as you get near the bladder in the lower abdomen.

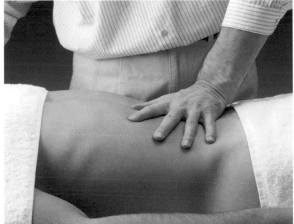

4 Do fanning, remembering that the impetus for the stroke comes from rotating the elbow. The hands and fingertips follow through, to give a mild friction/stretch to the abdomen. Repeat three times.

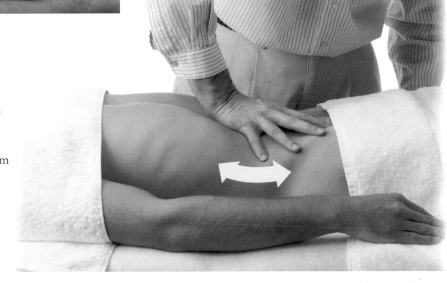

5 Apply a deep scooping effleurage from the lower to upper abdomen with outstretched fingers, 20 times. Owing to muscular antagonism this stroke is helpful with low back problems.

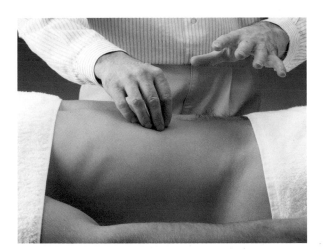

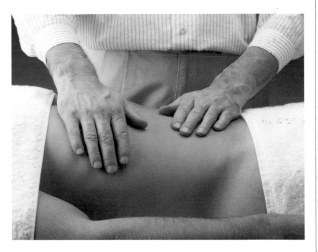

6 Perform picking up for 20 seconds. This stroke almost bounces on the abdomen and tenses the muscles. It can be disconcerting, so explain to your patient that it increases muscle tone. If the abdomen is well-muscled it may be appropriate to add hacking percussion.

7 Effleurage the whole abdomen smoothly but not too lightly, to complete the massage treatment. If any of the strokes in the sequence cause problems, experiment by practicing on your own abdomen to develop an acceptable touch.

CHEST MASSAGE

THE CHEST CONTAINS the muscles of the rib-cage, the shoulder, and the upper arm. At the front, a woman's sensitive breast tissue prevents massage of the pectoral muscles that draw her arms forward. Men can also find direct pressure on the front of the chest uncomfortable, so the chest massage described here combines circulatory movements with a gentle working of the muscles. When circulation gets congested here, some patients may find chest massage unacceptable. If so, try an alternative treatment using cupping percussion or friction generally over the ribs to help loosen up the congestion.

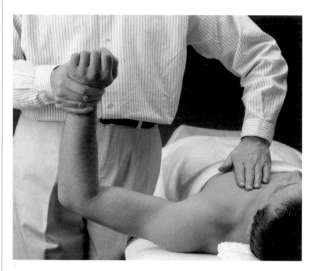

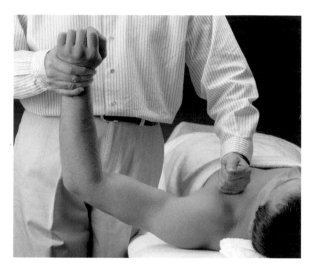

1 Hold the patient's arm at the wrist and draw it away from the body. Effleurage the arm with your inside hand, continuing the stroke to the shoulder, then glide along the chest just beneath the collarbone and on to the breastbone. Make the return stroke stronger toward the underarm, then lighter as you work back up the arm. Repeat six times.

2 Raise the elbow a little off the couch. Place the edge of a soft fist into the area where the chest, arm, and shoulder muscles merge. Make circular pressing movements for 20 seconds, then repeat the effleurage stroke.

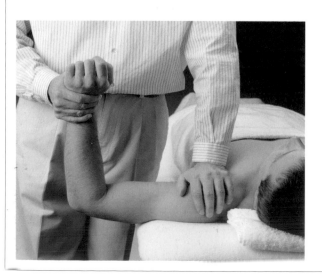

> **OPTION**
>
> Chest massage can be combined with strokes for the back if the patient lies on his side. It is then possible to treat half the back with the shoulders and rib-cage. This is the best position when using cupping percussion to relieve congestion.

3 Place the heel of your hand in the petrissage position and curl your fingers over the shoulder. Ask the patient to breathe in deeply. On the out breath, depress the shoulder and gently shake the elbow forward and backward. Hold pressure for five seconds. Repeat the effleurage and do the complete movements twice more.

NECK MASSAGE

ANXIETIES SEEM TO provoke tension in the neck more than anywhere else in the body, probably as an expression of defensiveness. Since this reaction does not facilitate problem-solving, tensions in the neck can become chronic. Fortunately, neck massage is very parasympathizing, which means that even the slightest contact has a direct influence on the neck nerves that unwind tension. As a result, most patients given neck massage would like it to last forever.

1 Place a small pillow under the patient's head, leaving the neck clear of the couch. Do light effleurage from the shoulders to the neck and face for 20 seconds.

PRECAUTION

An arthritic condition that affects the wrists or hands may damage the stability of the neck joints. In this case, a gentle version of neck massage can be done with the patient sitting upright.

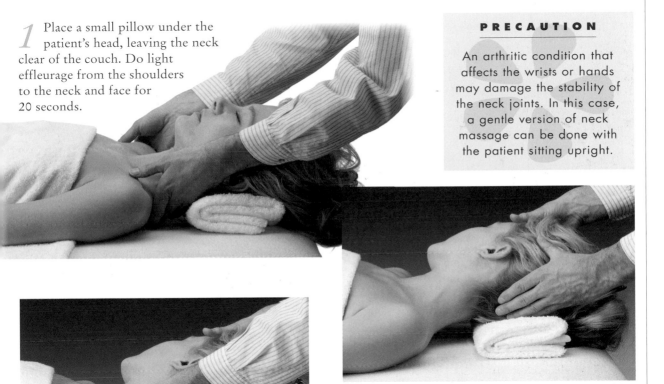

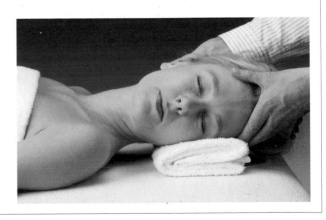

2 Roll the head a little to each side. Without lifting the head or twisting the neck, roll the head further to the right side.

3 Steady the forehead with your right hand. Using the edge of your left hand, petrissage the neck from the top of the shoulder to the back of the head, up and down six times. Do not press the neck with your thumb. Effleurage downward six times and repeat to the left side.

4 Lift the head clear of the pillow and rotate it to the left side. Try not to tilt or stretch the neck off-center. Looking at the neck, the slender rotation muscle on the righthand side should be aligned to the center of the body.

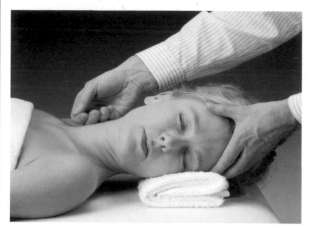

5 With curled fingers, stroke up and down the rotation muscle. It is sometimes very apparent, but, if not, move your fingers from just behind the ear to the center of the chest. Stroke for 20 seconds. Lightly effleurage. This is the most effective part of neck massage, but it does not involve more pressure than is needed for good skin contact. Lift the head clear and, after pausing for a moment in the center position, rotate it to the right and repeat the strokes.

6 With the head returned to center, do fingertip effleurage from the top of the arms to the top of the neck for 20 seconds.

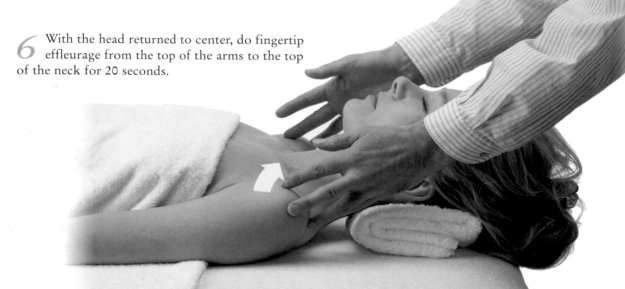

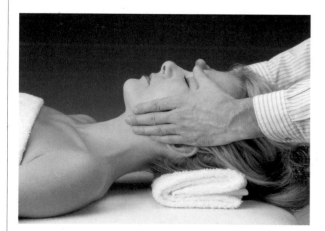

7 Make a smooth effleurage stroke from the neck to the face, widening the cheeks. Continue the stroke lightly over the ears.

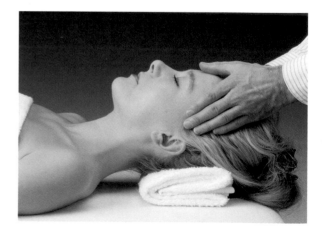

8 Begin a final effleurage from the top of the shoulders. Continue through the side of the neck, widen the cheeks and then, with thumbs extended, smooth over the forehead. Return to the shoulder via fingertips and repeat six times.

NECK AND FACE MASSAGE

ECK MASSAGE GIVEN in the sitting position has the advantage that pressure from tension is easily drawn downward. Because the patient retains some control of the neck muscles, the posture of the neck and head can be improved. This is one of the most pleasurable and spontaneous massage sequences, and it has inspired many skeptics to explore massage further and experience the benefits of whole-body treatments.

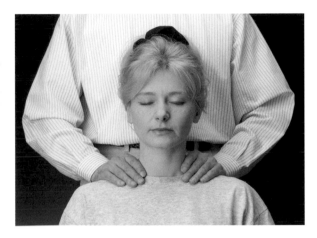

1 Standing behind the patient, do light effleurage from the sides of the head down the neck and over the shoulders to the upper arms. Repeat six times.

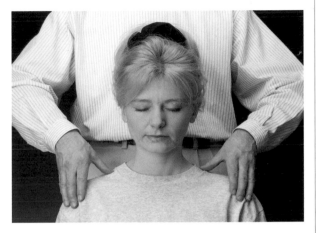

2 Do petrissage on the ridge of the shoulders. Use your thumbs, resting the fingers over the shoulders, moving from the center to the outside edges for 20 seconds. Effleurage as before.

3 Hold the forehead in the palm of your right hand and petrissage by lightly squeezing up and down the back of the neck for 20 seconds. Repeat on the other side. Effleurage as before.

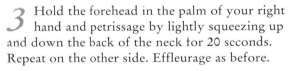

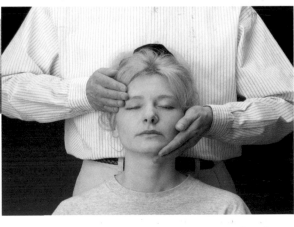

4 Stand close in and allow the patient's head to rest against your abdomen. Effleurage from the forehead to the temples, and from the chin to the temples, six times.

5 Petrissage for 20 seconds, using the fingertips to circle lightly over the face. Be very gentle near the eyes. Effleurage as before.

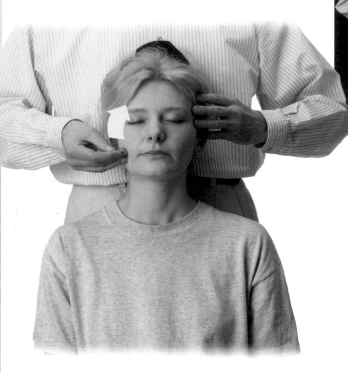

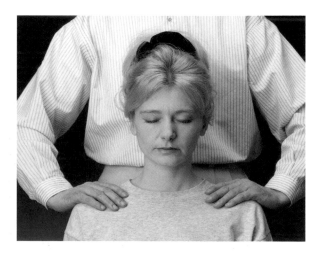

6 Use tapping percussion, with one fingertip after another, drumming all over the face for 15 seconds. Avoid the eyes and the tip of the nose. Effleurage again.

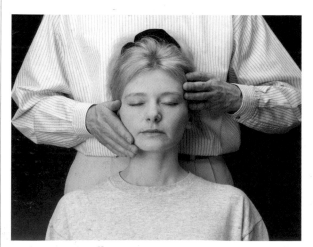

7 Gradually restore the head to the independent position but continue to support it with one hand. Effleurage one side, from the head through the neck and shoulders to the upper arm, six times. Repeat on the other side.

8 Ask the patient to begin supporting her neck herself. Effleurage, initially using alternate hands from forehead to shoulder, then double hands. Repeat six times. This stimulates the neck's postural muscles and helps recovery from what can be a very soporific massage.

COMPLETING THE MASSAGE

WHEN YOU COMPLETE a massage sequence, cover your patient with towels to keep the muscles warm and maintain his or her sense of being cared for. A massaged patient may want to talk, may be drowsy, or may even be asleep; you should be available during this time of transition back to normality, but you may feel the need to withdraw slightly for a few minutes while the patient readjusts. Professional practitioners recognize this possibility by giving a 50-minute massage in a one-hour treatment period, since this allows a few minutes for a satisfactory ending.

A MASSAGE CONCLUDES with a few moments' complete rest. Some deep breathing is often valuable at this stage. When your patient is ready to leave the couch, give support until he or she is safely upright. Some practitioners prefer to leave the patient to get dressed, but it is quite important to stay nearby to give attention or guidance if this is the person's first experience of massage.

Individual reactions to massage treatment vary, but in the short term most people feel a reduction of pressure and an increase in comfort. Some may experience mild disorientation, and a significant reduction in tension can lead to some unsteadiness. If this occurs, the patient will need to be reassured and given time to readapt. More commonly, your patient will enjoy the pleasant sensations of heightened physical and emotional awareness, and feel more integrated and energetic.

Positive long-term effects of massage are secured by regular treatments. Regular patients seem to recognize and appreciate the massager's touch with increasing contact, and this enables a deeper sense of relaxation to be explored. Improvements in postural misalignments or restrictions recorded at the initial sessions can also be confirmed during later sessions. The trust that builds up between patient and practitioner makes it easier for the patient to manage stress by responding sensitively to his or her own physical symptoms.

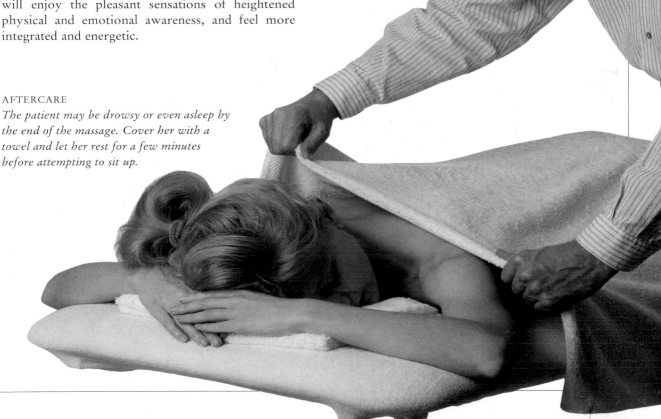

AFTERCARE
The patient may be drowsy or even asleep by the end of the massage. Cover her with a towel and let her rest for a few minutes before attempting to sit up.

MOBILIZING JOINTS

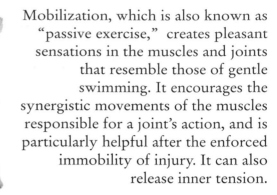

THE STROKES OF a massage treatment are complemented by stretching movements known as "mobilizing." These involve manipulation of the limbs so that each joint is flexed or extended as fully as possible, throughout its natural range of movement. This is done in cooperation with the patient, but without his or her conscious involvement.

Mobilization, which is also known as "passive exercise," creates pleasant sensations in the muscles and joints that resemble those of gentle swimming. It encourages the synergistic movements of the muscles responsible for a joint's action, and is particularly helpful after the enforced immobility of injury. It can also release inner tension.

ARMS AND LEGS

THE ARM AND LEG joints should be able to move very freely over a lifetime. Movement is normally initiated by nerve impulses to the muscles, but in mobilization the massager initiates and carries through the movement. If you are familiar with the anatomy of joints and take into account the patient's case history and normal range of movement, you can confidently apply such mobilizations. The following passive exercises can be safely practiced by keeping within comfortable limits of stretching. For maximum benefit, move the joint in an obvious direction up to the point of resistance, and just a little further.

JOINT FLEXIBILITY

Mobilization is all about increasing flexibility in the joints. Each of the major mobile joints in the body is a complex mechanism of articulated bones, cartilage, ligaments, and tendons operated by powerful skeletal muscles.

The knee, for example, is so important to the stability and locomotion of the body that it has 10 muscles passing over it and 10 ligaments holding it together. It looks vulnerable, yet it is the strongest of all the freely moving synovial joints. It does suffer when unexpectedly twisted, and sometimes the ends of its bones become painfully inflamed through the stresses of carrying an overweight body.

Such inflamed or swollen joints are not suitable for mobilization, since this may add to the problem, but if a joint is simply underused through inactivity it is sure to benefit from the sensitive stretches involved in passive exercise.

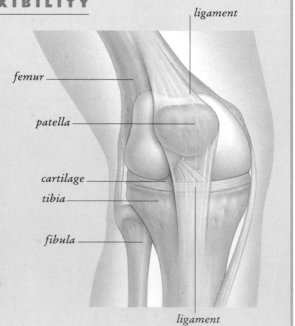

ligament

femur

patella

cartilage

tibia

fibula

ligament

Mobilizing the Arm

THE ELBOW JOINT forms a hinge, but it is also capable of a peculiar rotation that contributes to the flexibility of wrist and hand movements. Try unlocking a door without your elbow's cooperation. Unfortunately, both the elbow and wrist are vulnerable to impact, and the elbow can become fixed through not being sufficiently relaxed. Mobilization can help restore flexibility in both cases.

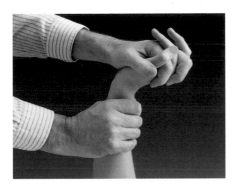

1 With the patient's elbow resting on the couch, fix the forearm, interlock the fingers and gently extend the wrist until you feel a soft resistance.

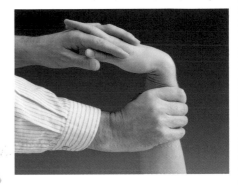

2 Slowly draw the wrist into flexion and stretch smoothly. Make sure you do not "bounce" the joint. Repeat these stretches.

3 Since the wrist is an "anglepoise" joint, mobilize it by moving it at random in all directions. Effleurage the wrist to complete.

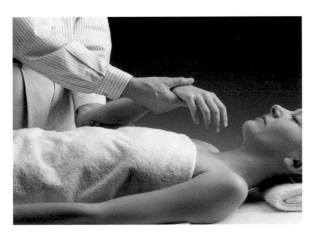

4 With the palm uppermost, support the elbow and flex to bring the hand toward the shoulder. Squeeze gently.

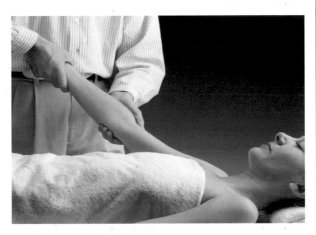

5 Extend the joint gradually and, when straightened out, softly stretch it a little further. Repeat the movements with the palm facing downward to fully mobilize the elbow.

Mobilizing the Shoulder

THE MOVEMENTS THAT the shoulder undergoes are usually very modest, considering its potential. It is unusual for anyone to raise their arms above head level, for example, and hanging by the arms is an activity restricted to the gym. In fact, our arms are better adapted for hanging than they are for lifting and carrying, and if they are not used in this way occasionally, the shoulders may need mobilizing to offset the pressures that build up through normal activities.

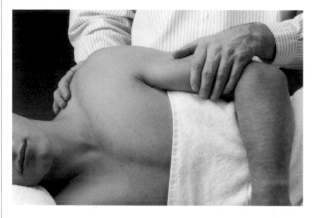

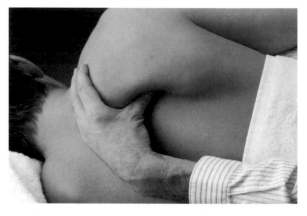

1 Place the patient in a sideways position and lay his arm along the side of his body. Steady the elbow and begin to loosen the shoulder by smoothly pushing forward and pulling back.

2 Define the scapula behind with your hands, and aim to get your thumb deeply underneath all along the edge of the bone.

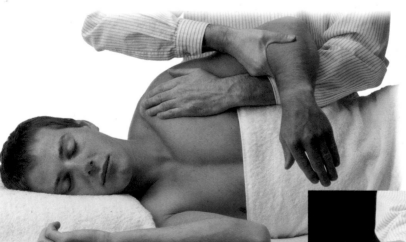

3 Lift the patient's elbow and thread your lower hand to the front of the shoulder. Move the shoulder up and down in the direction of the head.

4 Clasp the shoulder between your hands and rotate, beginning with small movements and increasing to involve the whole shoulder. Do rotations in the opposite direction. Then fold the arm across the couch on top of the other arm and cover to keep warm.

Mobilizing the Ankle

THE ANKLE JOINT is potentially extremely flexible, but since you walk around on one of its bones, the heel, the weight of your body alone is enough to stiffen it up. The problem is made worse by urban living, for the ankle does not appreciate the flat, predictable ground surfaces created by most civic authorities. Having evolved over millions of years to accommodate a wide variety of surfaces and pressures, the ankle is often desperate for some real movement.

2 Place your hand over the back of the foot. Make sure the leg remains passive at 90 degrees. Press down gradually to straighten out the heel with the rest of the lower leg over six seconds. Release, increase the stretch momentarily, and do effleurage.

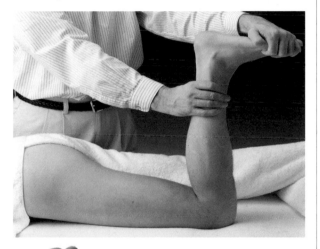

1 Passively flex the knee to 90 degrees. Steady the leg just beneath the ankle with one hand and hold the foot with the other. Check that the leg is still passive and slowly straighten out the ankle over six seconds. Release a little, then increase the stretch. Hold for six seconds. Release and do effleurage of the ankle, then repeat the movements.

3 After checking once more for position and passivity, explore each angle of movement by deliberately moving the foot around in the manner of a desk lamp, in any direction. Move it slowly, then a little quicker, first one way and then the other. Do firm effleurage to complete the mobilization.

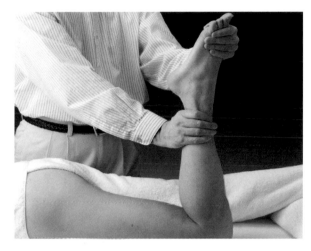

Mobilizing the Knee

THE KNEE IS THE largest joint in the body, which is just as well, since it has to accommodate the weight of the body bearing down from above it and the pressures and shocks of walking transmitted from below. Although protected from twisting by its ligaments, the knee suffers much of the strain of twisted posture, so it is important that the leg muscles are kept well-toned. Low back pain is often referred directly to just one knee, a fact that often baffles patients.

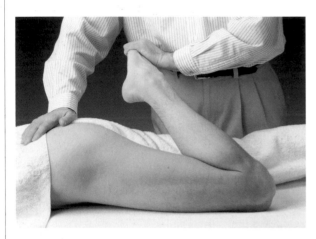

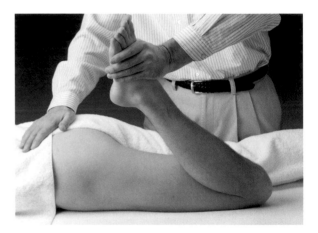

1 Place your right hand on the pelvis, reach over and flex the opposite knee to 90 degrees. Slowly fold the foot toward the opposite buttock until you feel a resistance. The pelvis should not move. Release a little, then increase the stretch for six seconds.

2 Bring the leg back to 90 degrees. Repeat the previous movement, this time aiming the foot to the outside of the left buttock.

3 Slide your hand into the back of the knee to make a soft wedge. Hold the foot and slowly stretch the leg onto the wedge. Pause when you feel a resistance, then stretch again for six seconds. Repeat twice more.

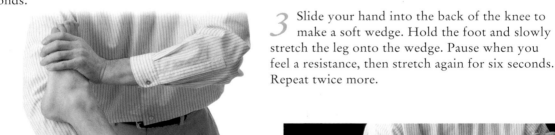

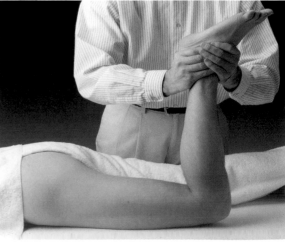

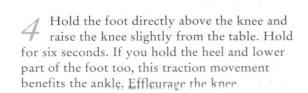

4 Hold the foot directly above the knee and raise the knee slightly from the table. Hold for six seconds. If you hold the heel and lower part of the foot too, this traction movement benefits the ankle. Effleurage the knee

Mobilizing the Hips

THE HIP IS A ball-and-socket joint, which makes it one of the most flexible in the body. Yet it often has to be surgically replaced, not because of overuse but through wear and tear that may be caused by standing immobile for long periods. Problems can also arise from sitting with thighs crossed on a chair, which strains the snugly fitting thigh bone from its socket. Mobilization can help limit such damage, and improves flexibility.

1 Stand close to the couch and hold the opposite leg at 90 degrees. Place your other hand on the pelvis. Check for passivity, then slowly draw the foot toward the other leg. The hip is being stretched when the pelvis tips up from the couch. Release a little, then increase the stretch for six seconds.

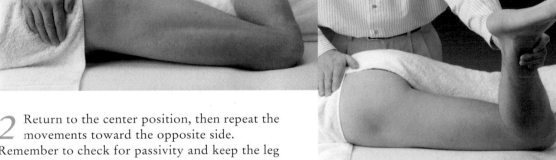

2 Return to the center position, then repeat the movements toward the opposite side. Remember to check for passivity and keep the leg at 90 degrees.

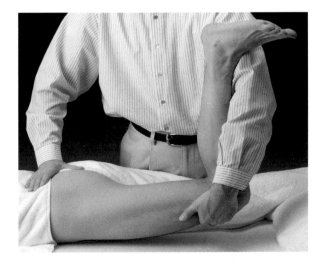

3 Feed your arm under the knee, resting the foot on your shoulder. Keep your other hand on the pelvis. Raise the knee so the pelvis begins to tip forward. Release, then increase for six seconds.

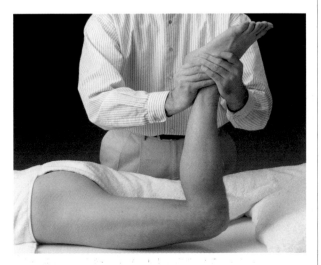

4 Hold the heel and foot to create a traction. Lift and lower slowly and swing from side to side. Transform this into a circling motion, both ways. Finish by effleuraging from knee to hip.

Mobilizing the Neck

THE NECK IS more mobile than the rest of the spine, but it does have the weight of the head to carry. Normally it achieves this gracefully, but tension in the shoulders can shorten the neck and restrict its mobility. If the head is thrown around in a fall or whiplash incident, the neck may be severely affected at the top, lower down where it joins the chest, and in the middle of its curve. It can take many years for the neck to recover its poise. Treatment to loosen muscle tension can relieve discomfort and pressure, but where the joints have become stiff, this mobilization can provide a painless release of deeper tension.

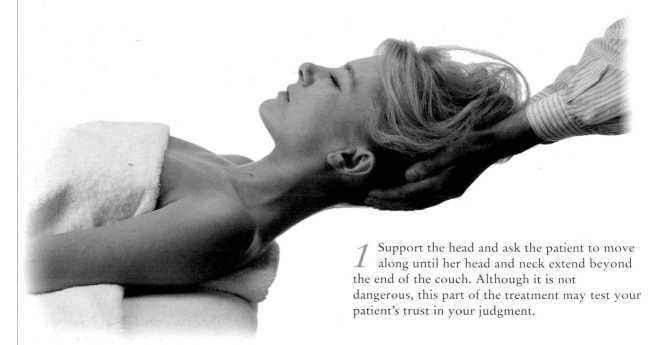

1 Support the head and ask the patient to move along until her head and neck extend beyond the end of the couch. Although it is not dangerous, this part of the treatment may test your patient's trust in your judgment.

PRECAUTION

Before giving this mobilization, familiarize yourself with the whole sequence so that you do not need to refer to the text. You can then give your whole attention to the movements.

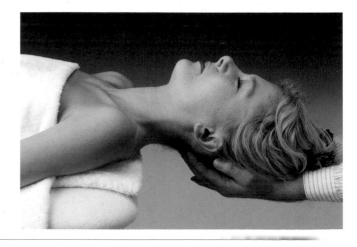

2 Beginning very slowly, lower the head and then raise it again a few times, until you feel the patient releasing control of her neck muscles. If you are successful you will feel the head become increasingly heavy.

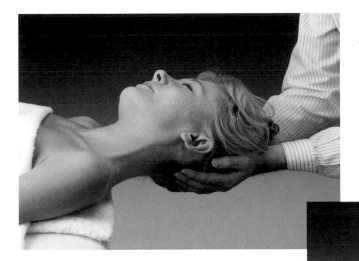

3 Move the head to each side in a tilting action, aiming the ear toward the shoulder. Repeat, moving it a little further the second time. Return to the center position and lower and raise the head once more.

4 Rotate the head slowly to the left. It is important to keep the neck in the midline. Pause for a few moments, then return to center. Repeat the sequence to the righthand side.

5 Rotate again to the left side. Lower the head a little, then a little more, and hold it quite still. This is the most helpful movement, so the head can be lowered as far as possible. Repeat to the righthand side.

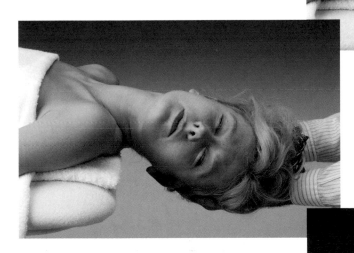

6 After returning to center, the whole treatment can be done again, when the patient's muscles are usually found to be more cooperative. With the head fully supported, ask the patient to move slowly back down the couch. Place a small pillow under her head.

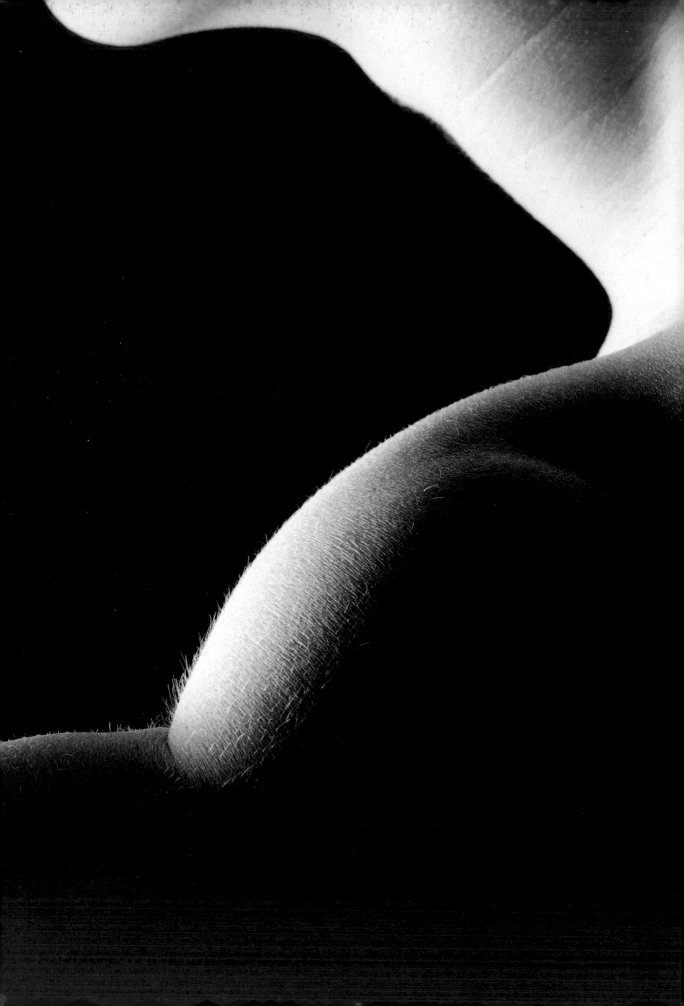

SPECIAL TECHNIQUES

THE HANDS-ON approach of massage has formed the basis for many special approaches and techniques. Some were developed long ago, and have evolved in parallel with basic massage therapy. Others have been devised quite recently as variations on the massage theme. These techniques are often mysterious, glamorous, or personalized, and this image has tended to cast doubt on their validity as effective therapies. Yet many patients have found that special techniques consistently relieve problems that do not respond to other treatments, and many professional massagers employ them as part of their daily practice.

SPECIAL APPROACHES AND TECHNIQUES

SHIATSU

Is Japanese-style massage. It is a pressure-point technique based on a concept of physiology similar to that employed in acupuncture.

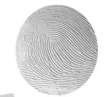

HYDROTHERAPY

Is massage using applications of water. It is most effective when the body is unable to tolerate hand pressure, and is consequently the first form of massage to be applied after injury.

AROMATHERAPY

Involves massage with highly aromatic plant oils. The use of the oils can enhance the effects of massage, and is particularly effective in releasing emotional tension.

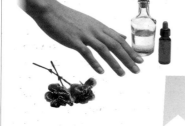

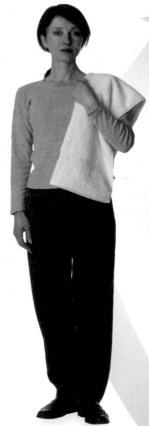

REFLEXOLOGY

Is one of the most ancient forms of massage therapy. I a micro-massage system, using pressure on the feet and hands influence the wellbeing of oth parts of the body.

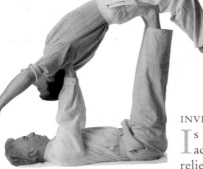

INVERSION THERAPY

Is a novel technique that combines basic acrobatics, yoga, and massage. Inversion relieves spinal pressure and the force of gravity is reversed, enabling massage to be given with great delicacy.

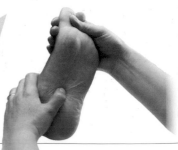

AROMATHERAPY

AROMATHERAPY INVOLVES massage using oil that has been blended with the essence of a plant. The essences themselves are a little oily, very fragrant, and usually too concentrated to be used neat. They have been used therapeutically since biblical times, and are extracted by a variety of methods according to whether the fruit, leaf, or stem of the plant is used. Vast amounts of raw materials are required to produce even small quantities of essential oil, and their harvesting and lengthy production make them expensive.

ESSENTIAL OIL MASSAGE has become a very popular therapy. It is esthetically very pleasing, and it has a scientific profile that has helped to raise its popular status more than regular massage. Several large pharmaceutical companies are undertaking research at the moment into the anti-bacteriological properties of essential oils, and if the results are encouraging they could represent an important step towards more ecologically sound medicines.

The attractive perfumes of essential oils have a measurable influence on the brain. Psychological studies have shown that scent is capable of adjusting a person's mood, and it is this quality that makes aromatherapy effective. By blending an essential oil with a base massage oil, or conducting massage in an

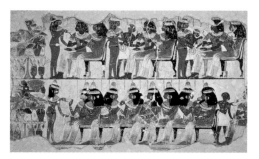

Natural fragrances have been valued for thousands of years, and were used for healing in ancient Egypt.

aromatic atmosphere, the effects of massage can be intensified. Furthermore, because the brain reacts to the stimulus of scent at infinitesimal levels, the oils can be used at very subtle doses.

Among the most sedative oils are those of sandalwood, marjoram, geranium, and bergamot. Stimulating effects are achieved with oils of basil, orange blossom, and Ylang Ylang. Jasmine flower oil has the same stimulatory power as caffeine, but has a negligible influence on heart rate.

Aromatherapy is based on superficial strokes, with the emphasis on assisting lymphatic drainage with various effleurages. There are moments when massage slows down and almost ceases, but despite this the effects can be profound and long-lasting.

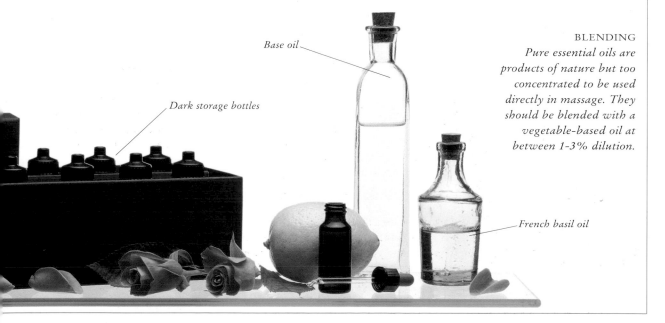

Base oil

Dark storage bottles

French basil oil

BLENDING
Pure essential oils are products of nature but too concentrated to be used directly in massage. They should be blended with a vegetable-based oil at between 1-3% dilution.

Aromatherapy Face Massage

CONSIDERING THE IMPORTANCE of its functions and musculature, the face is a strangely neglected area. A treatment of the face is a micro-massage that achieves a whole-body effect through nervous feedback from the facial nerves to the autonomic nervous system. This interrupts the cycle by which anxiety produces facial distortion, which in turn maintains anxiety. The essential oil used should have an affinity with the skin and parasympathetic nervous system, but always check your choice with the patient.

1 Stand or sit at the patient's head within easy reach of her face. A towel or headband can be used to hold the hair back. Apply a small amount of oil to your hand: try lemongrass at one percent strength, in grapeseed oil.

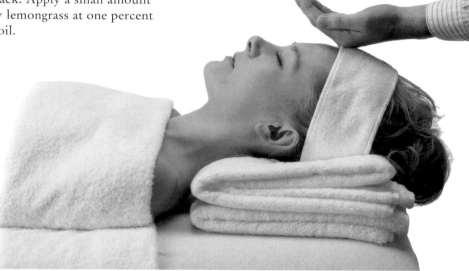

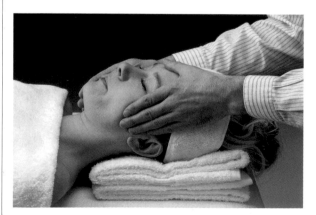

2 Pause to let the oil take up the temperature of your skin, then begin effleuraging the face from the chin to the temples and across the forehead, 10 times.

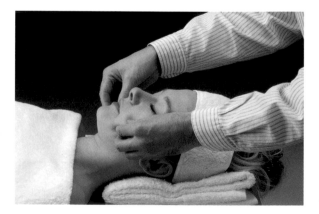

3 Do circling strokes with your fingertips on the cheeks: from the chin toward the ears, nose and eyes, for 10 seconds.

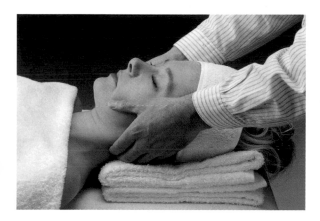

4 Effleurage toward the ears with the outside edges of your thumbs six times, then repeat the strokes.

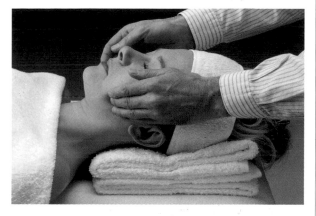

5 Perform light petrissage along the jaw to its hinges by the ears. Reverse the stroke and, on reaching the chin, continue petrissage around the mouth, moving the lips but without opening the mouth. Repeat three times. Effleurage toward the ears six times.

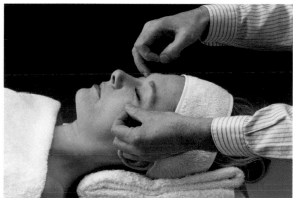

6 Using the middle finger, firmly effleurage the upper rim of the eye socket, from center to temple, six times. Do the same to the lower rim with the thumb.

7 Be aware of tension lines on the forehead – horizontal, vertical, or both. Apply friction with the middle fingers at right angles to the lines for 20 seconds. Effleurage the temples and hairline six times. Repeat the strokes.

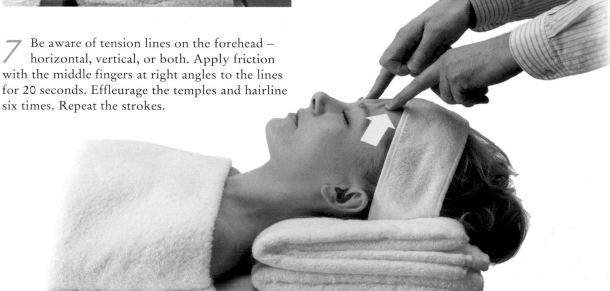

8 Hold the ear lobes and pull gently down and away from the head, either independently or together, vibrating for 10 seconds.

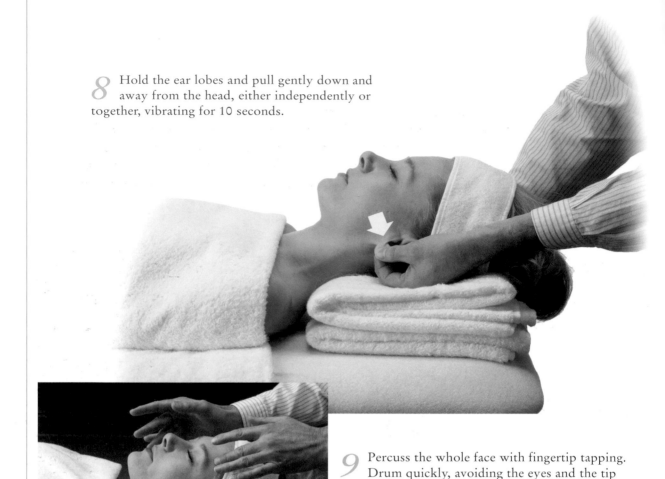

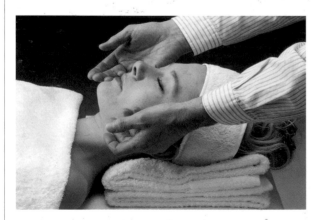

9 Percuss the whole face with fingertip tapping. Drum quickly, avoiding the eyes and the tip of the nose, for 20 seconds.

10 Slowly effleurage the face from the chin to the temples and across the forehead 10 times, using a steadily lighter touch as you finish the strokes.

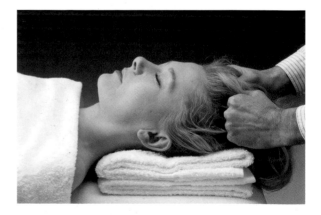

11 Comb through the hair with your fingertips, lightly scratching the scalp. Take good handfuls of hair and squeeze and pull until the scalp stretches, three times. It is best not to stroke the face after working on the hair, so finish by effleuraging the shoulders.

Aromatherapy Back Massage

AN AROMATIC BACK MASSAGE can be a profound experience. A wide variety of invigorating strokes can be applied to the skin, and these have a stress-relieving influence on the nervous system through reflex action. The oily medium of the massage enables even the most tender back muscles to be treated delicately and sensitively. The essential oils chosen for back massage may reflect a circulatory or topical affinity with the body.

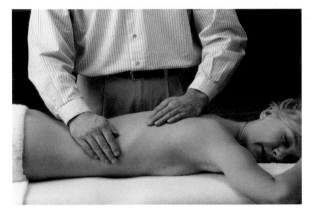

1 Before applying the oil, friction the whole back with your palms and fingertips to increase the circulation to the skin.

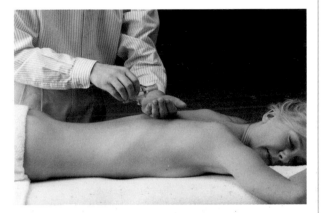

2 Rest your hand on the patient's back and pour a teaspoonful of oil into your palm. You can add more oil during the treatment as necessary. A good choice for this treatment is sandalwood in sweet almond oil.

3 Do effleurage across the whole of the patient's back. This will spread the oil evenly, but do not expect it to give a "slippery" feel.

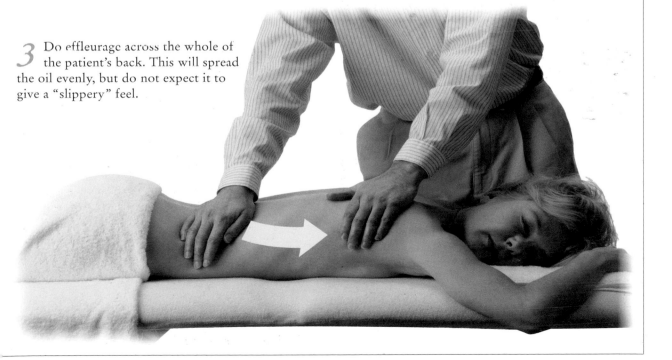

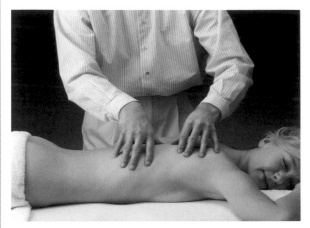

4 Perform raking for 20 seconds. Concentrate on the rib-cage, then effleurage all across the back and repeat the movements.

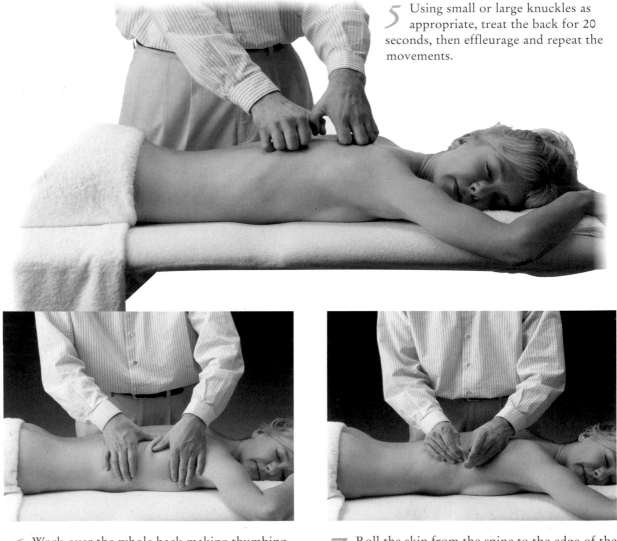

5 Using small or large knuckles as appropriate, treat the back for 20 seconds, then effleurage and repeat the movements.

6 Work over the whole back making thumbing stretches of the skin and underlying tissues, then effleurage and repeat.

7 Roll the skin from the spine to the edge of the chest and from the shoulders down to the pelvis. Effleurage and repeat.

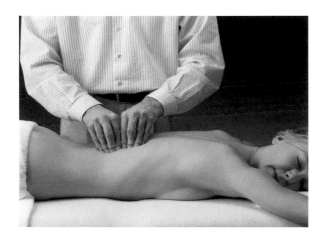

8 Do petrissage to either side of the spine, from the back of the neck to the sacrum, and return. Effleurage and repeat the strokes twice.

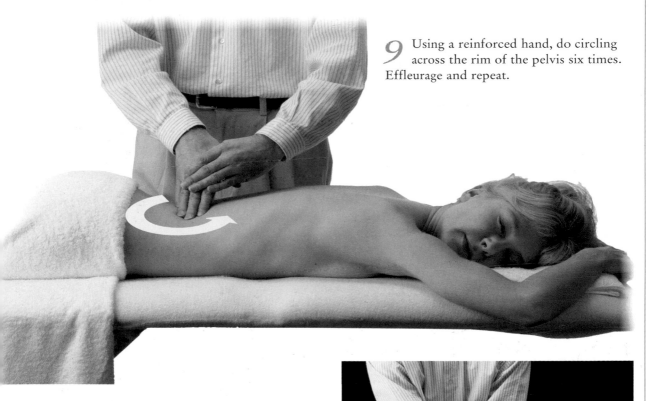

9 Using a reinforced hand, do circling across the rim of the pelvis six times. Effleurage and repeat.

10 Make a final deep effleurage, sweeping across the length of the back while interchanging your hands, from shoulders to pelvis. Reduce pressure, slow down, and end by trailing your fingertips lightly over the back. Cover the patient and allow a few minutes more recovery time than with regular body massage.

SHIATSU

SHIATSU IS A JAPANESE massage system derived from Chinese theories about how the body works, using concepts of energy to describe its therapeutic benefits. Although differing in minor ways, shiatsu technique is rather like acupuncture using the fingertips instead of needles. The strokes are aimed at points on the skin that are said to be the focus of pathways associated with the working of the internal organs. A shiatsu practitioner concentrates spiritually on his or her own abdominal center, the "hara," while the hands are located on the patient's energy points.

SHIATSU FOLLOWS THE tradition of other Oriental therapies in that, ideally, it is a preventative technique. Many Japanese use the services of the visiting shiatsu therapist for regular treatment, and family members also practice on each other.

Shiatsu is a very safe and environmentally friendly massage therapy, because it requires no equipment or technology and is usually performed on the floor. This allows very direct pressure to be applied to the body, and is also advantageous to the practitioner, whose posture is considered important to the transmission of healing energy. The patient may not have to remove any clothing, and simply lies in a comfortable position. Treatment sessions tend to follow the intuition of the practitioner, who works from the hara.

Sometimes shiatsu is reported as being painful, but since the strokes are not particularly deep, the discomfort probably arises from congestion of the pressure points, implying overwork. When this is the case, the therapist will usually suggest ways of improving lifestyle and habits. Shiatsu practitioners do take a case history – as do other professionals – which screens out any patients who are unsuitable for full-scale treatment. At home, apply the rule of always massaging within comfortable limits.

Shiatsu is regularly used for problems associated with fatigue and exhaustion. It is known to exert a calming influence, while, conversely, those who feel low report that it has an energizing effect. Many people find the technique useful for acute pain relief in the joints, and also find that it helps with long-standing posture problems. Shiatsu practices have also been integrated into novel Western techniques such as the "Seated Massage Experience." This involves taking massage to the patient's workplace for mid-morning or mid-afternoon sessions, echoing the way shiatsu is traditionally practiced in the East.

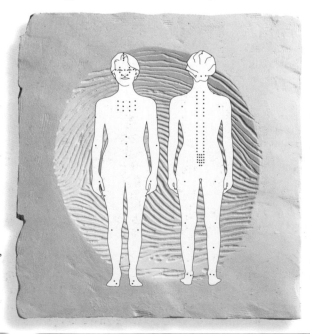

Shiatsu is based on a "subtle" Oriental anatomy of energy pathways linking the body's organs, which can be treated by pressure-point techniques.

Shiatsu for the Shoulder

SHIATSU SPECIALIZES in pressure-point application, and is usually recommended for both acute and chronic conditions when other massage techniques fail to trigger a healing response. An immobilized shoulder is typical of the problems than can be treated in this way. Patients having shiatsu for the first time should have the technique explained in advance, to maximize cooperation with breathing and prepare for the sensation of the pressure stroke.

1 Stand behind the seated patient and ask for a mobility demonstration of the shoulder. After effleurage, steady the body with one hand while gently probing the shoulder area for tender points with your fingertips. There are often unexpected areas of tenderness.

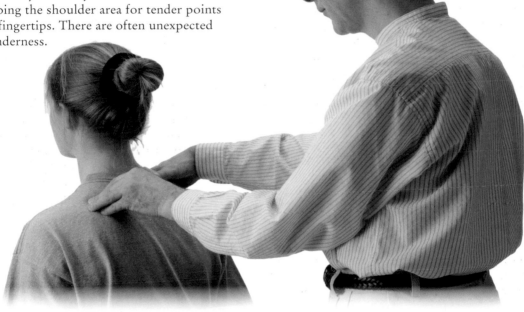

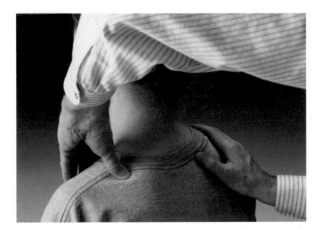

2 Place your thumb directly over a new point. Ask the patient to breathe in deeply and exhale slowly. On exhalation, apply pressure to the muscle beneath. Slowly release on inhalation and effleurage the point with small circling movements.

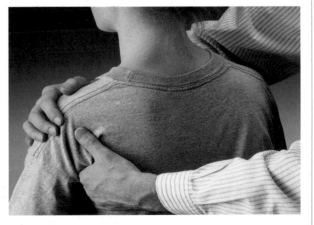

3 Treat other similar points in the shoulder in the same way, using both thumbs one on the other if necessary, then apply deep effleurage. Test the extent of active shoulder mobility again and note any changes.

Shiatsu for Fatigue

MOST ORIENTAL CULTURES share a physical and spiritual regard for the feet that goes far beyond the concepts of care accepted in Western countries. In the East, the feet are revered as a sacred part of the body, partly because they represent our contact with the earth. Foot massage is particularly valued as the perfect preparation for sleep. The technique described here is recommended for fatigue and exhaustion, and demonstrates the therapeutic use of the feet in shiatsu.

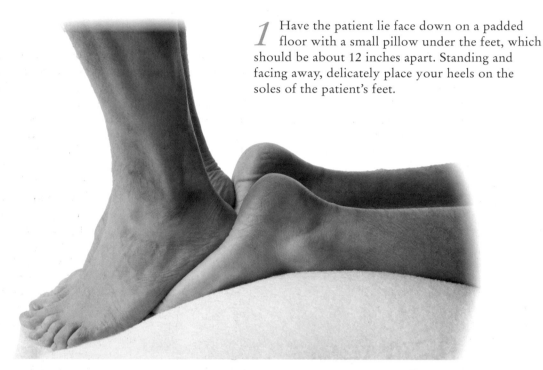

1 Have the patient lie face down on a padded floor with a small pillow under the feet, which should be about 12 inches apart. Standing and facing away, delicately place your heels on the soles of the patient's feet.

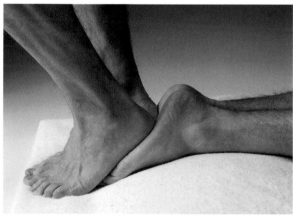

2 Keeping your knees slightly flexed at all times, gradually apply your full weight to the patient's feet. Transfer your weight rhythmically from the left foot to the right by increasing the knee bend one leg at a time.

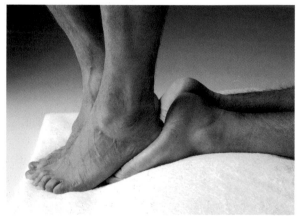

3 Obtain deeper pressures by straightening the knee and focusing contact through the heel. Treat the whole foot for up to 10 minutes. If the patient's foot suddenly cramps, then stop, extend the big toe, and effleurage the instep.

HYDROTHERAPY

HYDROTHERAPY IS massage treatment using water. It is the most commonly applied form of massage worldwide, yet most people who use hydrotherapy are not aware that they are practicing it. They simply know that water is a great healer of aches and pains, strain and tension. All life begins in water, so hydrotherapy reconnects people with a naturally life-giving and healing environment. The body's physiological response to water gives this form of massage a particularly valuable role in the treatment of illness and the management of injury.

THE CLINICAL USE of hydrotherapy was developed in nineteenth-century Europe from techniques used in folk remedies. A Silesian farmer called Preissnitz is credited as the pioneer in this field, but the most famous early hydrotherapist was Sebastian Kneipp, a Bavarian priest. Kneipp avoided an early death by embracing hydrotherapy, and later became an internationally renowned healer.

Kneipp's followers have succeeded in bringing the traditions of hydrotherapy into the modern era, and there are numerous well-documented examples of its effectiveness in pain relief, as a reliable sedative, and in the restoration of healthy circulation.

It is not difficult to explain how hydrotherapy works. Being warm-blooded, the human body benefits from contact with cool water; briefly applied, the water acts as a tonic, while extended applications have a calming effect.

Contrasting hot and cold applications are also used and, occasionally, longer hot applications. Hot hydrotherapies are versatile in that they can be anti-inflammatory when placed in opposition to an injury. Applying heat to an unharmed leg, for example, diverts blood toward the treated area and reduces the blood's pressure in the injured leg.

The influence of hydrotherapy is initially recorded in the skin and then distributed throughout the body via the nervous reflexes and circulatory routes. The water is administered by various methods ranging from splashing to immersion, as well as moist compresses. Hydrotherapies are suitable for patients of all ages, and are particularly valuable in cases of infirmity and chronic illness. Hydrotherapy is also very effective when used on children, who both benefit from the treatment and actively enjoy it.

HEALING WATER
Water is universally valued for its soothing, relaxing qualities and its natural healing power. Hydrotherapy simply builds on the benefits that everyone enjoys through contact with clean, fresh water.

Hydrotherapy for Muscle Spasm of the Calf

THE CIRCULATION IN THE LEGS sometimes has local difficulty meeting the needs of hard-working muscles. This can cause cramp, a painful and often briefly incapacitating problem that, if occurring regularly, needs investigation. This can be supported by a specific hydrotherapy treatment using water of contrasting temperatures. The therapy has a gentle yet penetrating action that encourages more efficient circulation, and works well on spasm of the limbs generally.

1 Have one bowl of very hot water and one bowl of ice-cold water near the treatment couch. Soak a face flannel in each. Apply the wrung-out hot cloth to the calf for 30 seconds.

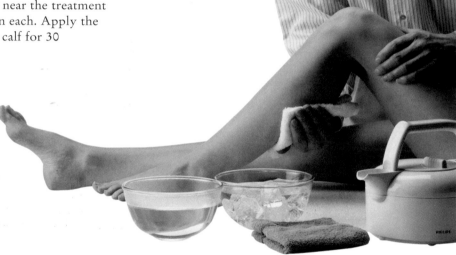

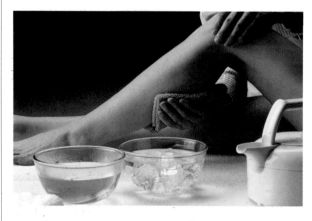

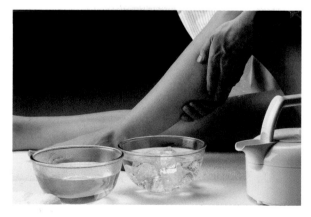

2 Replace the cloth in the hot water and apply the cold flannel for 30 seconds. Repeat six times, hot and cold, re-soaking the cloths between applications. Keep a kettle nearby to top-up the hot water, since the used flannel will cool it.

3 Effleurage the leg deeply, from ankle to knee, 20 times. The arrangement of this hydrotherapy massage sequence allows it to be carried out as a self-treatment if necessary.

Hydrotherapy for Varicosity of the Lower Leg

IF BLOOD RETURNING from the leg meets with resistance higher up in the body, a vein in the leg may stretch to accommodate the pressure, causing a varicose vein. The flow may be obstructed by pregnancy, constipation, low back, or pelvic tension, and any treatment to help recovery of the vein must take these factors into account. Hydrotherapy is an effective relieving treatment, but should be combined with back and abdominal massage to ease the strain on the veins.

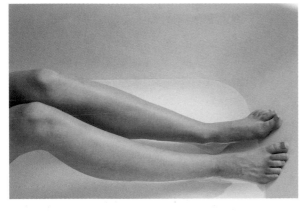

1 The patient should sit in a warm bath with her legs out of the water, resting on the end of the bath or on a comfortable support.

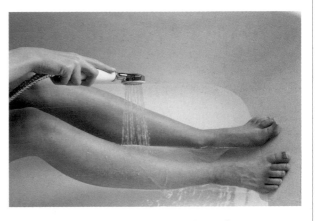

2 Play a cool hand shower or jug of water over the leg from the ankle to the knee, but not back down, 12 times. Repeat the cool-water sequence with the other leg.

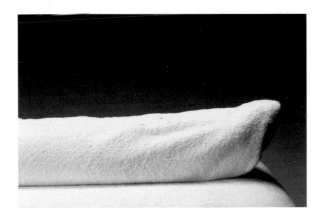

3 Allow the bath to empty. When the patient leaves the bath, she should dry her body but simply wrap her legs in a towel.

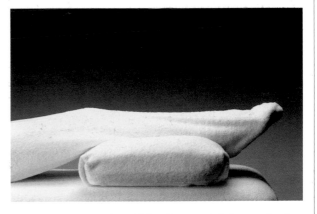

4 The patient should lie down with legs raised and supported by a pillow for 10 minutes. This hydrotherapy makes a very worthwhile self-treatment.

REFLEXOLOGY

REFLEXOLOGY HAS a long pedigree. Its techniques were practiced during the ancient Egyptian and Chinese civilizations, while its recent history is related to twentieth-century zone therapy. It is based on the idea that massaging reflex points on the feet and hands can influence distant parts of the body. The reflexes extend from the extremities to the top of the head, along "meridians" or pathways, and influence the vital organs in passing. By applying finger pressure to the reflex points, the reflexologist aims to release energy in the meridians, which decongests, invigorates, and helps maintain a balanced state of health.

TWENTIETH-CENTURY reflexology was pioneered in the United States by Dr. William Fitzgerald, a medical practitioner who had previously worked in Vienna. While there he came into contact with the European tradition of pressure-point massage, and was able to show its anesthetizing effect for minor surgery. Although his ideas were not well received in general by his professional colleagues, Fitzgerald gained an enthusiastic follower in Dr. Joseph Riley, a general physician. Riley's interest was shared by his assistant Eunice Ingham, who clarified our present-day understanding of the reflexes. Her unique contribution was to create the functional mapping of the feet that is familiar to all contemporary reflexologists.

The feet, hands, and ears have all been proposed as mapped areas for reflexes. If the trunk and head are projected onto the soles of the feet, the head is

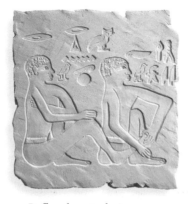

Reflexology techniques were practiced by the ancient Egyptians over 3,000 years ago.

represented at the toes with the abdominal cavity at the heels. The instep of each foot acts as a reflex for the spinal column, while the limbs are represented as folded along the outside of the foot. The ear is, in effect, the patient as a fetus, shown upsidedown, so that the earlobe represents the skull, and the rim of the ear represents the spine.

Reflexology is an evolving therapy that is establishing itself as a gentle, noninvasive technique. Its positive philosophy makes it an attractive preventative therapy, and many patients have found it useful for coping with chronic conditions and systemic disorders related to hormonal functioning. It has been used palliatively in conventional healthcare and has been favorably received among the nursing profession in particular. It has the advantage of being complementary to other therapies, and there are no side effects attributed to it.

REFLEXES
Although reflexology can be practiced on various parts of the body, such as the hands and ears, it is the feet which are regarded as the most receptive areas for treatment.

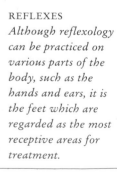

Reflexology for the Back

REFLEXOLOGY CAN BE used to treat the back when acute muscle spasm makes it impractical to apply a direct treatment. This is particularly true of problems in the upper back and neck region. It is also possible to use reflexology to assess back problems when sensations of pain are ill-defined or very extensive. In such cases, the spinal points are examined generally and any tenderness or pressure felt is related back to the muscles of the spinal column.

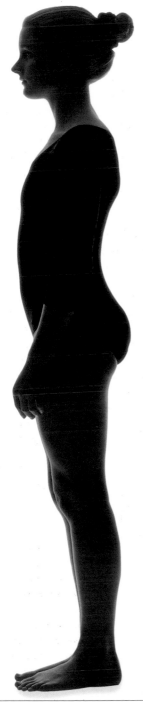

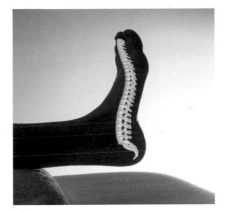

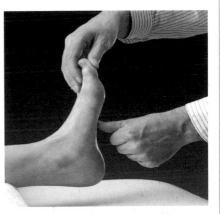

1 Ask the patient to stand side-on, facing left. Note the spinal curvature. Ask the patient to lie down and view the left foot from the right side to compare its silhouette with the spine. Individual curves may match, if not the whole curvature.

2 For treatment, place a pillow under the knee and ankle so that the foot is extended. Steady the foot by lightly holding the toes, and effleurage the instep with the edge of your thumb, with even pressure in both directions.

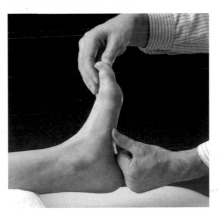

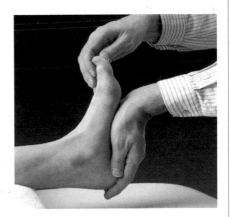

3 Using a pointed edge of the thumb, trace along the instep, sensing for hard contacts. These points are usually deeper areas of pressure in the back muscles. Treat them with gentle effleurage circling using a flatter part of the thumb, for up to two minutes each.

4 Complete the treatment by effleurage, using the whole hand. Wrap the foot in a warm towel and repeat the whole procedure with the other foot.

INVERSION THERAPY

INVERSION THERAPY is a very advanced technique. It is not dangerous to perform, but it must be learned through personal contact and under the close supervision of an instructor. For this reason the description given here is purposely incomplete. It is not a step-by-step instruction sequence but merely an illustration of the range of positions that are involved in this radical new therapy.

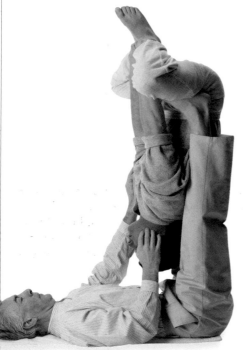

Inversion therapy, originally known as "acrosage," was developed by Benjamin J. Marantz, who became a student of massage after a professional career in acrobatics. As he studied, Marantz became aware of a relationship between the two activities. He realized that, in supporting his acrobatic partners, he had been unconsciously activating pressure points similar to those described in shiatsu.

This observation became the basis of inversion therapy. It involves the practitioner using his legs to support the patient upsidedown while leaving his arms free to massage the upper body, especially around the face and head. Mobilizations can also be given to the spine and limbs, and the patient may be allowed to simply relax in the inverted position.

The technique is claimed to be very safe and suitable for most people, except those who have serious cardiovascular problems or medical conditions of the eye. Marantz himself explains its advantages in terms of the reversal of gravitational forces, which relieves pressure on the spine and congested areas of the body such as the lower abdomen.

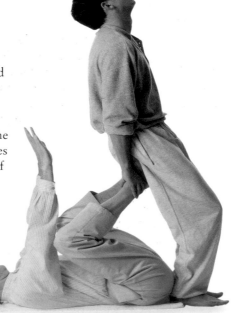

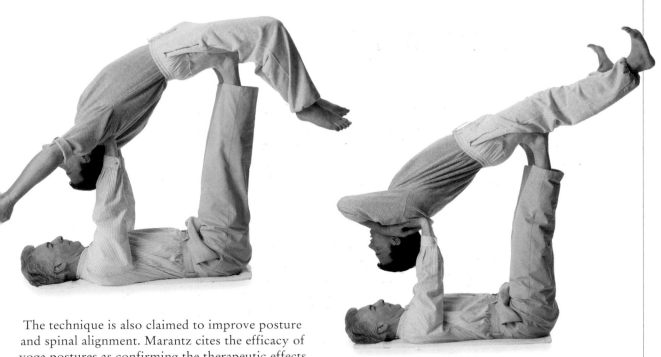

The technique is also claimed to improve posture and spinal alignment. Marantz cites the efficacy of yoga postures as confirming the therapeutic effects of inversion, and considers that the supporting technique central to his therapy makes it accessible to people with spinal or neck disorders. He believes that inversion therapy also boosts self-confidence and quotes this as the most common psychological response to treatment.

Inversion therapy is consistent with many other forms of massage in that it is also beneficial to the giver. The technique does not depend purely on strength, and when perfected it can be given to a patient of up to twice the therapist's body weight.

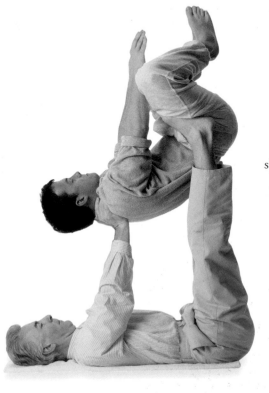

Using muscle control and the structure of his or her own skeleton to support the patient, the practitioner can relax freely while massaging, and feel refreshed on completion.

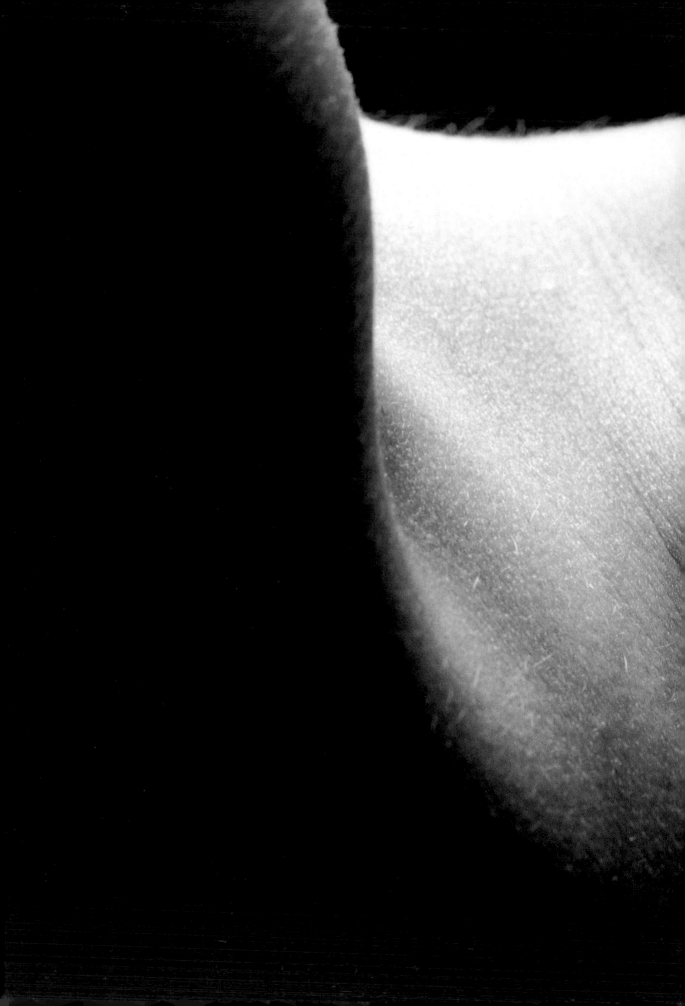

Special Treatments

MASSAGE FOR PREGNANCY

THE PSYCHOSOMATIC NATURE of massage therapy makes it a beneficial
form of care during every stage of pregnancy. It helps to condition both
the body and the emotions during the prenatal stages, relieves both pain
and alarm during labor, and helps ensure rapid postnatal recovery.

THE CHANGES IN the body that are brought about by
pregnancy are, of course, primarily for the benefit of
the baby. In this sense, the mother accommodates the
baby at her own physical expense, so it is
understandable that, for the majority of women, the
lengthy preparation for birth is a physically
strenuous experience.

Pregnancy can also be psychologically taxing. The
excitement is accompanied by apprehension about
the outcome: the baby's health, the possible pain and
danger of childbirth, and, even if it is not the first
baby, the unknown future. It is a time, therefore,
when sensitive emotional support is as important as
proper physical care.

If the balance of care is inadequate, this failure is
reflected in pressure rises in the mother's body,
particularly in the cardiovascular system. Blood
pressure can rise dramatically, and the veins –
particularly those that carry blood returning from
the legs and pelvis – commonly become distended.
Although normally classed as disease symptoms,
such conditions are really indicators that the level of
care is insufficient. In general, pregnancy seems to
give some protection against true diseases;
established conditions such as arthritis often abate
for the duration of the pregnancy and reappear only
after the birth.

It is very important that physical prenatal care,
while screening for any medical problems that would
endanger the pregnancy, takes into account the
unnatural effects of modern living on the body. The
flexibility and endurance upon which successful
pregnancy and birth depends often has to be
specially developed – a fact that is recognized in the
prenatal programs that prospective parents are urged
to attend. Massage can be of great value here. It can
also help relieve tension during the birth itself, and
dispel the fear that has been identified by many
observers as a significant factor in complicating
normal delivery.

POSTNATAL CARE

Once the baby is born, the body obviously has to
accommodate to the trauma of having given birth.
Even the most straightforward birth results in
serious injury, of a nature which, if received in a
sports activity, would command close attention.

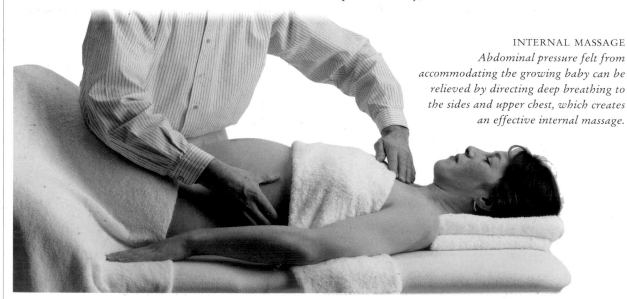

INTERNAL MASSAGE
*Abdominal pressure felt from
accommodating the growing baby can be
relieved by directing deep breathing to
the sides and upper chest, which creates
an effective internal massage.*

Unfortunately, the mother's well-being is often assessed simply in terms of survival, while the baby becomes the center of attention. If the signs of injury are ignored, subsequent pregnancies may run into complications, and, in the longer term, the mother's general health may be disturbed. Well-judged massage therapy can help prevent such problems.

The physical trauma of birth is at least obvious, even if its consequences are sometimes ignored. It has only lately been recognized, however, that giving birth may be emotionally wounding even if the physical outcome is satisfactory. The emotional damage may arise from the unique experience of pain, the sudden implications of parenthood, or, perhaps, the mother's association with the pain of her own birth. Getting appropriate psychological help at this time may be even harder than obtaining physical therapy, because it is generally assumed that motherhood should produce a surge of happiness. The reassuring touch of massage may be just what the mother needs to heal the damage and prepare her for her new role.

Leg Massage for Pregnancy

IT IS IMPORTANT to massage the legs from the earliest days of pregnancy. Any postural problem tends to become magnified in pregnancy, and back problems, particularly, can refer pain to the legs. It is also a time when tiredness begins to show in the legs, and massage is a way of ensuring that the patient gets some rest. This is even more essential for pregnant women who are already parents.

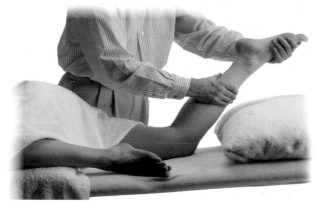

1 Have the patient lie face down on the couch with one leg drawn up and the knee placed on a pillow to accommodate the abdomen. Effleurage the lower leg.

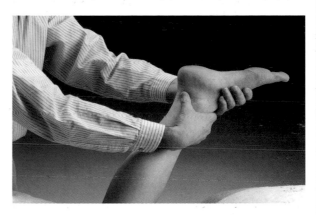

2 Give frictions encircling the ankle and a little way up the lower leg for 30 seconds. Use moderately deep strokes, avoiding any indication of varicosity.

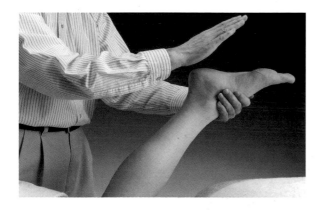

3 Apply percussion generously to the sole of the foot, tapping with all your fingers.

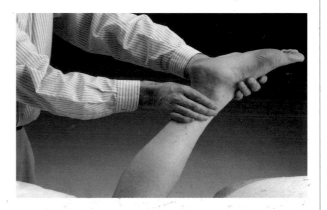

4 Give slow, deep effleurage up the leg from the foot to just beyond the knee.

Abdomen Self-Massage During Pregnancy

A MODIFIED FORM of abdominal massage is valuable during pregnancy. The simplest effleurage strokes can be used at first, then easing pressure strokes as the baby develops and the mother's muscles start to take the strain. It is important that the mother chooses which strokes feel most helpful and how long the massage should last, and for these reasons, self-massage is often a good option.

1 The patient should lie on her back with her legs raised on a pillow. The whole of the abdomen is effleuraged with soft rolling strokes, defining its shape and lightly stretching the skin.

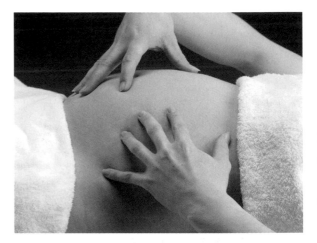

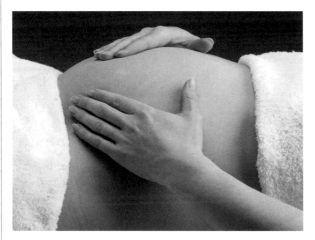

2 Using a modified raking stroke, the outstretched fingers and thumb are drawn around the abdomen. This can also be done as a light, rhythmic scratching, to include the waist.

3 Beginning wide at the sides, the hands are slowly pressed against the waist muscles and slid inward, gradually releasing pressure toward the center of the abdomen. In late pregnancy, when it is less comfortable to lie on the back, the strokes can be done seated.

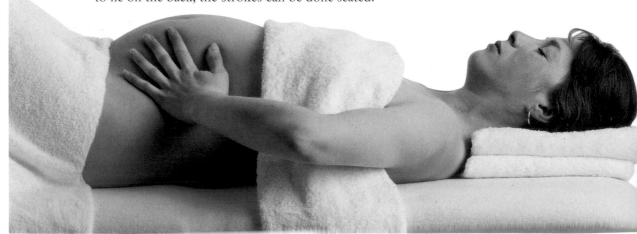

Back Massage During Birth

BACK PAIN DURING LABOR is caused by the pelvic adjustments needed to allow birth, as well as pressure build-up in the muscles. This discomfort can be difficult to ease, but walking around, having a warm bath, and deep breathing are all known to offer some relief. Massage aims to help by using the principle of counterirritation, so the strokes are begun quite vigorously – in fact, many patients ask for the power of the strokes to be increased during labor.

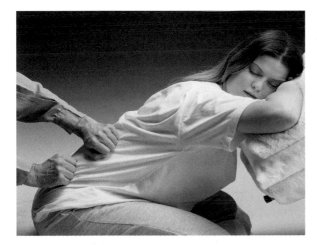

1 Ask the patient to take up a kneeling position, leaning forward with her legs apart. If kneeling is not comfortable, try a standing position, leaning forward on a support.

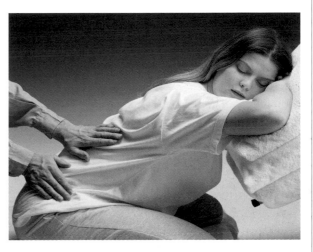

2 Leaning her upper body forward takes the weight off her spine. When her shoulders are relaxed and her jaw muscles are released, give smooth effleurage to her whole back.

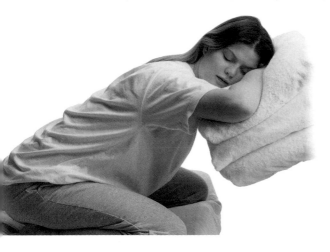

3 Use your knuckles to petrissage the shoulders and lower back. Pay particular attention to the pelvic area. The strokes and varying pressures can be rehearsed throughout the pregnancy to prepare for the day when they are needed.

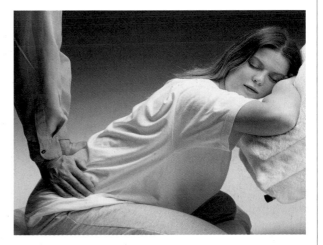

4 Placing your hands on either side of the pelvis, give a strong downward pressure as the mother breathes out. Repeat, taking care not to overstretch the legs.

MASSAGE FOR BABIES

W HEN A BABY is born, it leaves a familiar world of massage and hydrotherapy and is ejected into a situation where human contact may be denied completely. In some cultures, newborn babies – especially males – are immediately separated from their mothers for extended periods, because such intimacy is thought to reduce the child's aggressiveness. Thankfully, this notion has not become widespread, and does not deter most parents from caressing, handling, and otherwise massaging their babies – providing, of course, they themselves have been similarly treated.

THE RELATIVE HELPLESSNESS of a baby invites loving hands, and the obvious delight, reassurance, or consolation that passes between parent and child confirms its naturalness. It is an interaction from which parents derive immense pleasure. When there is unforeseen separation, as when babies are born preterm and have to survive in an incubator, the parents suffer obvious distress; clinical findings suggest that the baby is badly affected too, and thrives better when even minimal physical contact is included as part of treatment.

Cradling a baby may be instinctive for most parents, but deliberate massage is only normal in certain cultures. In India, babies are massaged for the first time six days after birth, and then daily up until the age of three. Weekly massage then forms part of nourishment and nurturing for the rest of childhood. In Western countries, by contrast, children usually receive massage only if it is medically indicated as a response to illness, rather than as part of maintenance and prevention. With just a little technical encouragement, reinforced by natural parent-child responsiveness, the lives of all babies could be enriched by regular massage.

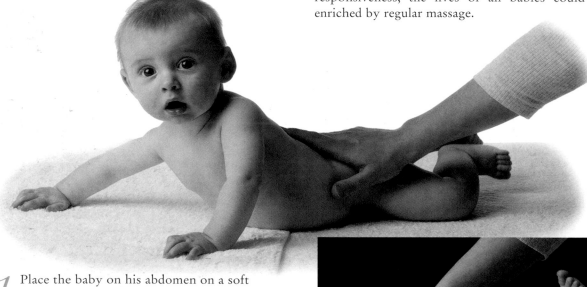

1 Place the baby on his abdomen on a soft towel, and allow him to settle. A nearby musical toy may help hold his attention. Place a soft palm on his lower back. Allow him to move or wriggle under your hand, then effleurage across his buttocks and up to his shoulders.

2 Roll the baby onto his back. Hold his foot in one hand and wring the leg from the thigh downward, three times. Repeat to the other leg.

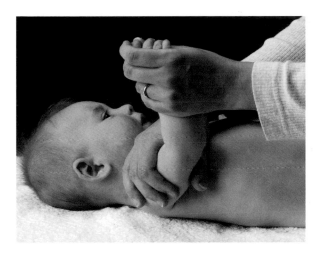

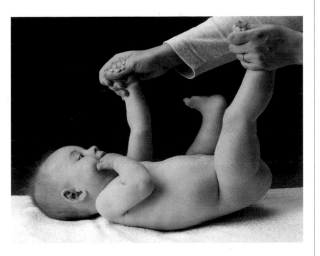

3 Draw his arm away from his body. Wring the arm from shoulder to wrist, three times. Repeat to the other arm.

4 Hold the opposite hand and foot. Draw the limbs toward one another and open them out again. Lift to straighten the limbs and gently resist the baby pulling away. Repeat to the other side.

5 Contain the baby's head with your hands and effleurage his forehead with your thumbs. This may calm the baby, or encourage more wriggling.

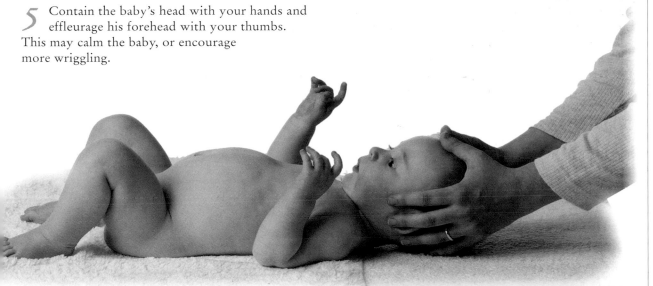

6 Continue effleurage to his ears, pinching lightly. Do circling on his forehead, temples, and scalp. Do whatever the baby cooperates with – a baby massage is treatment at its most interactional! Don't expect to complete a whole sequence at one massage session, and vary the order of strokes according to the baby's response.

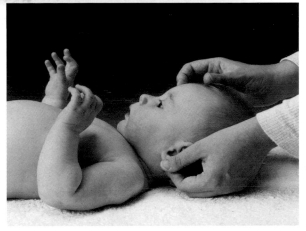

MASSAGE FOR CIRCULATION

MASSAGE IS PREEMINENTLY a muscle therapy, but it can also improve the efficiency of the circulation systems. There are three of these in the body. The nervous system circulates information to and from the brain, and in the process it organizes the fluid circulation; this is subdivided into the bloodstream and the lymphatics. An understanding of the lymphatic system is crucial to an appreciation of the role of massage. Older adults especially benefit from circulatory massage.

DRIVEN BY THE pumping action of the heart, blood is forced out through arteries of ever-diminishing diameter, to reach every cell of the body. The cells take up oxygen and nutrients from the blood and exchange them for carbon dioxide and other waste products. These are then delivered back to the heart in the returning blood, through the venous system. The right side of the heart pumps this venous blood to the lungs, where the carbon dioxide is replaced with oxygen. The refreshed blood then returns to the heart's left side, from where it is pumped around the body again.

As the blood interacts with the cells it loses some of its water content (plasma), and this produces a fluid environment for the body. If the fluid loss were to go unchecked, however, the body would become "waterlogged." To prevent this, the free water is claimed by the lymphatic system, and this lymph is recycled back into the bloodstream.

The lymphatics achieve this by channeling lymph along vessels that lie almost in parallel with the veins. In fact the lymph vessels share many physical characteristics with the venous system, and the two types of vessel converge just before the heart so that

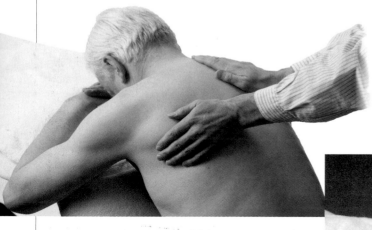

1 For the head and neck: have the patient sit facing the back of a chair leaning over against a pillow, making sure that the head and neck are well supported. Effleurage the whole back.

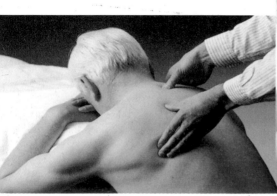

2 Use raking, thumbing, and knuckling to petrissage the chest and shoulders. Begin lightly and increase in depth and speed.

3 Use your thumbs to gently press along below the skull and down either side of the neck. Do light effleurage down to the shoulders. Ask the patient to breathe deeply three times, to complete the massage

lymph enters the whole blood just in time for re-circulation. Because the lymph contains white "disinfecting" cells and can become impure, the system is filtered on the way to the heart. The filters are called nodes (or, mistakenly, "glands") and when they are especially active they raise their temperature to add a combustion effect. This is when we become acutely aware of their presence as "swollen glands" in the joints and at the base of the skull.

To understand how massage can help optimize this system, it is important to realize that while the heart actively pumps the blood out, it cannot suck it back. Returning blood and lymph is propelled along by the alternating contraction of the skeletal muscles, the pressure against the skin created by firm contact (as when walking), and by the rhythm of breathing.

Venous blood finds it easier to return than lymph, since it is in a closed circuit; movement of the lymph relies more on the tone of the muscles, to the extent that a well-toned body is capable of recycling 300 percent more lymph, per day, than an unfit body. It is the sluggishness of lymphatic return which gives a slack body its characteristic swellings, mainly around the ankles but also as puffiness in the face.

Lymphatic massage has been developed to assist with this problem. It is not possible to greatly speed up the lymph flow manually, but massage is able to relieve congestion and normalize the conditions upon which lymph flow depends. The massage is slow, and involves gentle rhythmic movements, since the skin itself can swell with lymph and may be easily injured.

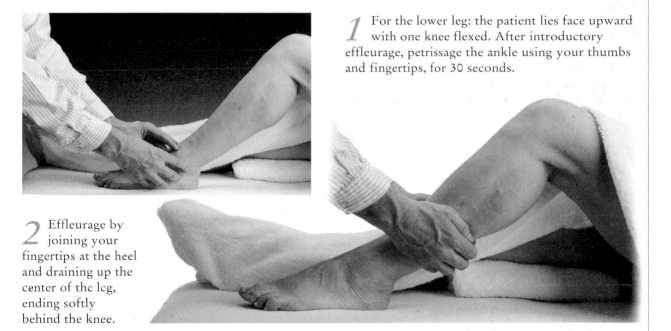

1 For the lower leg: the patient lies face upward with one knee flexed. After introductory effleurage, petrissage the ankle using your thumbs and fingertips, for 30 seconds.

2 Effleurage by joining your fingertips at the heel and draining up the center of the leg, ending softly behind the knee.

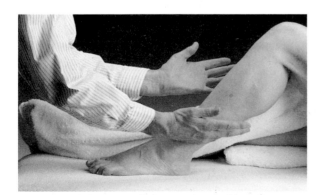

3 Do fanning by alternately sweeping your fingers up from the heel to either side of the back of the knee. Begin slowly, then slightly increase speed, up and down, for 20 seconds.

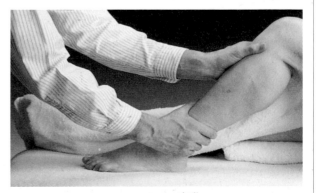

4 Effleurage firmly upward from the front and back of the leg, carrying out the stroke six times with each hand. Circulatory massage strokes may require a little oil on an older skin.

MASSAGE AND INJURY

MASSAGE HAS A VALUABLE role to play in helping the body recover from injury. Many injuries affect the muscles directly; the manipulations of massage stimulate the self-repair processes of those muscles and help prevent the complications that can arise from immobilization. Massage also stimulates the circulation, facilitating the delivery of vital nutrients and the removal of breakdown products. The movements of massage can provide a form of physiotherapy for stiff and damaged joints, and when bones are broken, massage provides valuable therapy for damaged soft tissues.

INJURIES ARE PART of everyday life: they record our overexertions. Some injuries are insignificant. Others, such as bone fractures, are major inconveniences. Sometimes we don't notice injuries, as with those bruises which can't be explained. Other injuries can be traumatic, in that our consciousness registers a reaction to any assault; when we experience such trauma, we are said to be in shock.

We usually make spectacularly complete recoveries from our injuries, and may marvel at the body's powers of self-repair. Even the most

devastating injuries are self-repairing, given minimum caring circumstances. By the time you are aware of a cut to the skin, for example, your body has already begun its repairing process. Few medicines have any positive influence on injuries, and a fractured bone – although sometimes requiring the skill of surgery for alignment – heals and makes itself stronger without any further attention.

The first way to deal with injuries is to prevent them, and this involves being careful – and thoughtful – about how we use our bodies. All too

DAMAGE AND RECOVERY

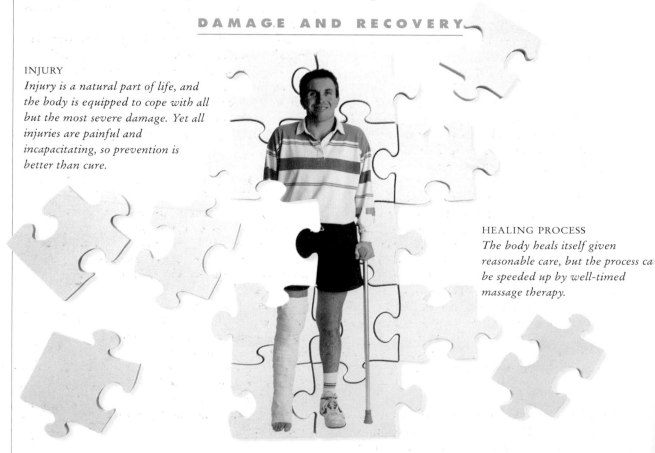

INJURY
Injury is a natural part of life, and the body is equipped to cope with all but the most severe damage. Yet all injuries are painful and incapacitating, so prevention is better than cure.

HEALING PROCESS
The body heals itself given reasonable care, but the process ca be speeded up by well-timed massage therapy.

LIFESTYLE DANGERS

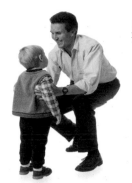

FAMILY LIFE
Most injuries occur in the home, possibly because we are off our guard in relaxed surroundings.

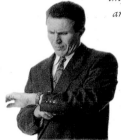

SPORTS
Physical exertion carries obvious risks, but these can be minimized by improving fitness and taking basic precautions.

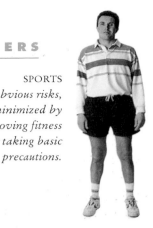

TENSION AND STRESS
Pushing yourself too hard dulls the reflexes and makes the body vulnerable to damage.

often people engage in strenuous physical activities when their bodies are not up to the job, and the injuries we call "accidents" are the inevitable result.

Some people seem to suffer injury more than others. Indeed, many injuries can be seen to have had a certain predictability. Unfit bodies cope less well with strain; tiredness and tension make us vulnerable to even minor exertion; an unbalanced diet can lead to weakness; carelessness often invites self-damage.

Preparing for physically demanding activities by doing regular exercise can help a great deal, and you should always do warmup exercises before any form of sports. Regular massage can help by keeping you supple and detecting and treating muscular problems before they cause trouble.

HOW TO AVOID INJURY

Our injuries possibly teach us more about ourselves than our illnesses do. Our experience of illness, in general, reinforces the idea that we have been the victims of bad luck. Our experience of injury is far more positive, since it teaches us either to avoid such situations in the future, or prepare for them.

One way to prevent injury is to face positively the prospect or likelihood of being injured. To this end, treatment that we know produces reliable healing can be modified and used regularly as a preventative. This follows a traditional edict in natural therapy: "the care is the cure and the cure is the care."

This approach allows you, as a massager, to offer massage with the emphasis on the containing, mobilizing, and supportive elements of injury treatment. These methods are best learned on uninjured partners, so that you develop confidence for dealing with injuries when they arise.

FITNESS

It is hard to find a definition of fitness with which everyone agrees. The condition of your lungs and heart are certainly relevant, and their performance can be assessed as a measure of fitness. Whether "more is better," however, is a debatable point. As long as you have a reasonable level of fitness, you will be protected from most forms of injury caused by sheer physical inadequacy.

TIREDNESS AND TENSION

These can be two sides of the same coin, suggesting strain and pushing up to and beyond tolerable limits. Sometimes it would appear that tiredness is offered as a sign of commitment to professional objectives, yet there is no doubt that our reflexes and reactions are dulled by excessive tension.

Those who are unscathed by going all out may succeed by making distinct changes in direction – they work hard, play hard, collapse, and bounce back again. This is effective, perhaps, but in ways most other people find too demanding – and too dangerous. Pushing yourself beyond your normal limit is a sure way of incurring injury of some kind.

WARM UP, WARM DOWN

Any physical exercise can injure your joints, muscles, and tendons. If you leap straight into action from rest, your blood flow rate does not have time to catch up; the muscles fail to work properly and are easily overstressed.

You can prevent this by warm-up exercises, which get the blood flowing well before you start working hard. After running you may also need to "warm down," which involves stretching muscle fibers that shorten as a result of repeated similar movements, causing loss of flexibility.

TYPES OF INJURY

OUR REACTION TO being injured often relates to how much inconvenience
it creates, as well as how much pain. For treatment purposes, injuries can
be categorized into two groups: "trivial" injuries, where the damage is slight and a
full recovery comes spontaneously through simple resting; and "serious" injuries,
in which there is destruction or discontinuity of tissue, resulting in temporary, or
even permanent, disability. Serious injuries often require medical intervention,
which can be incapacitating in itself, and massage therapists spend a lot of
time dealing with such problems.

INJURIES ARE OFTEN considered trivial because of the
situation in which the injury occurs, rather than the
damage done, since we tend to assume that an injury
is insignificant if it has a trivial cause. In these
circumstances, people are surprisingly ready to
trivialize quite painful, incapacitating injuries.

A truly trivial injury is not always easy to assess;
usually there is mild stiffness and some
inflammation, but if this diminishes after 24 hours
we feel a recovery has been made. Many trivial
injuries are caused by overuse of the body, and a
degree of interruption and rest will usually keep
problems at bay, even if the work has to be taken up
again later. If this fails, the injury will probably recur
again and again; such recurring injuries, like the
common bad back, require careful investigation –
both of the condition itself and of the circumstances
that provoke it.

MORE SERIOUS INJURIES

Trivial injury can sometimes develop into serious
injury, but in most cases pain, swelling, or loss of
blood will make any severe damage apparent from
the outset. A serious injury need not, of course, be
life-threatening: a vigorous reaction to the injury
actually demonstrates that the body is in full, healthy
response. However, a serious injury will require
more time to heal, and this provides an opportunity

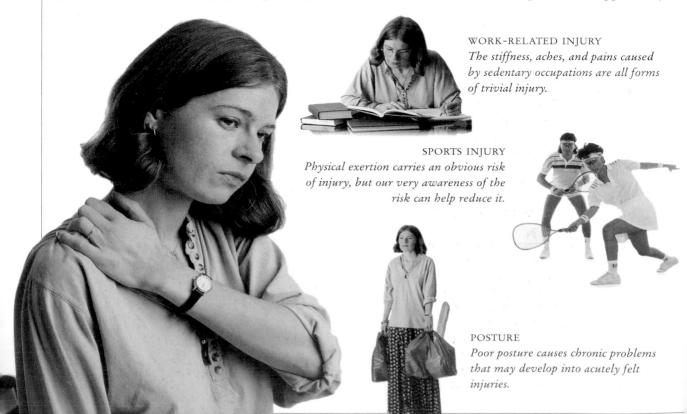

WORK-RELATED INJURY
*The stiffness, aches, and pains caused
by sedentary occupations are all forms
of trivial injury.*

SPORTS INJURY
*Physical exertion carries an obvious risk
of injury, but our very awareness of the
risk can help reduce it.*

POSTURE
*Poor posture causes chronic problems
that may develop into acutely felt
injuries.*

to apply appropriate treatments to optimize the body's effort. Specialized massage techniques have much to offer in these cases.

HOW THE BODY RESPONDS

The body's response to injury is commonly seen as a process of destruction, but this is only true if some serious disorder such as necrosis sets in. With most injuries the destructive phase is over very quickly, and once the injury site has stabilized, the body begins the process of repair. This may be painful, and we naturally regard pain as a negative quality, yet in truth it is proof that the tissues are vibrant and active.

Injuries almost always involve loss of blood, since tiny blood vessels are easily ruptured. The escaping blood seeps between layers of body tissue and is further distributed by the effects of gravity. This can explain why a bruise does not always correspond with the painful area. If a significant portion of circulating blood is lost, this can cause a major disturbance in blood pressure, which is often more serious than the initial injury.

Soon after injury has occurred, the small vessels begin to constrict and the blood clots. This is achieved by the coagulating cells in the blood – the platelets – which, along with the fibroblasts or matrix cells, link body tissue back together again. Providing that the injury is not aggravated, all this happens quite quickly.

While the injury is in the initial stage of blood loss, the undamaged, adjacent blood vessels dilate and allow blood that is more fluid than usual to arrive at the injury. This blood is called "exudate," and contains an increased number of the white blood cells called leucocytes, which attack any foreign matter in the injury. The exudate is very effective in disinfecting the injury, helping to stiffen the area and inhibit movement that would complicate the damage. It also stimulates the growth of new tissue.

Heat, redness, swelling, and tenderness all indicate exudation. Considering the value of such a spontaneous response, these secondary pains should be borne bravely, but massage intervention can alleviate much of the discomfort.

THE BODY'S RESPONSE

Damage to the delicate blood capillaries of the body caused by the wear and tear of life is continually repaired without disturbing the way they function. During injury, however, a mass of blood is lost, and this makes an integral "first aid" response necessary. A major feature of this is increased fluidity around the injury, for example from lymphatic swelling around a joint, which helps deal with inflammation. This contributes to the pressure on the nerve endings which results in pain.

HYDROTHERAPY

It is important to contain an injury, and the wisest method is to mimic the body's fluid response by using hydrotherapy. As soon as possible after the injury occurs apply cool water, either by immersion or by bandaging. This therapy can be used throughout the course of treatment to control pain. Flowing effleurage strokes are the most appropriate form of massage, while rehabilitation exercises are more beneficial when done under water.

BLOOD LOSS

EXUDATION

INFLAMMATION

PAIN

CONTAINMENT

THERAPY

REHABILITATION

TREATING COMMON INJURIES

THE CONTRIBUTION MASSAGE can make to the healing process has long been appreciated by athletes and dancers, who regularly sustain muscle injuries that require rapid and effective therapy. Yet massage can help with a far wider variety of common injuries, ranging from minor strains to major bone fractures. Some problems may need conventional treatment before massage can be of value, while others may respond to massage therapy immediately. In most cases, though, the right form of massage applied at the right time can be immensely beneficial.

MOST MASSAGE CONSULTATIONS take place when the acute phase of injury is over, after some form of diagnosis and initial treatment has been given. The conventional treatment may have been carried out by a surgeon, or by a physiotherapist using ultrasonic treatment to restore functioning. When massage therapy follows such initial treatment, it complements the orthodox approach by supporting the innate healing tendencies within the body.

There are also occasions where massage offers an alternative to orthodox therapy. This is most effective when the basic requirements of injury management are not being fulfilled by conventional methods, commonly in the early and late stages of recovery. Massage can be given in the form of delicate hydrotherapy at the beginning of a treatment program. It can also be employed in the later rehabilitation stages, when it is valuable because it

does not introduce overexercise without adequate rest. Another advantage of massage therapy is that it does not underestimate the emotional trauma caused by injury. The fact that the massage is given by the same therapist throughout each phase of treatment helps with psychological as well as physical recovery.

The gentle approach of massage as an injury therapy is based on the pattern of recovery from injury that operates in childhood. At this time the body is very efficient at repairing damage, and a child is more likely to express pain and receive emotional support, and is able to rest more than an adult.

Massage therapy can supply the same needs and help restore some of the recovery potential we all had as children. Given the enormous recuperative powers of the human body, appropriate massage has the potential to raise an injured adult to a higher state of fitness than he or she enjoyed before the injury.

THE REFERRAL SYSTEM

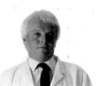

SURGEON
Injuries are usually attended to by surgeons, who are experienced in assessing the extent of damage. Most common injuries benefit from hydrotherapy massage as soon as possible after diagnosis.

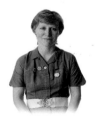

NURSE
Nurses are increasingly being given responsibility for treating minor injury and are using independent massage practitioners in rehabilitation programs.

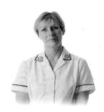

PHYSIOTHERAPIST
The expertise of the physiotherapist is perfectly complemented by therapeutic massage, since the two types of therapy share many common aims.

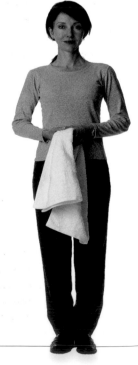

MASSAGE FOR FRACTURE

Abone fracture is one of the most serious disorders of the body. The muscles, nerves, and other adjacent organs are often incapacitated, and it can involve major blood loss. Since the bones are the body's framework, the entire skeleton has to adjust to accommodate one fractured bone. Yet despite these complications, bone fractures are rarely life-threatening unless the bones of the spine or skull are involved.

FRACTURED BONE TISSUE heals well, although not as fast as commonly believed. Limb fractures that are freed from their casts after six to ten weeks are not quite healed; it is simply that movement and pressure are required to continue the healing process. And the broken bone itself is only part of the problem.

Bones break only under exceptional pressures, by which time other, more elastic tissues will have been taken beyond their limit. The ligaments, whose role it is to guard against such eventualities, will have been stretched to the point of sprain. The muscles will have been pulled and severely strained. Meanwhile, the skin and other connective tissues with sensitive nerves will have been shocked. Conventional treatment tends to ignore this damage to the surrounding tissues – damage that can leave a fracture site vulnerable to inflammatory conditions in the long term.

First and foremost, the plaster cast, while effectively immobilizing the injury, does not offer appropriate treatment for the traumatized softer tissues. All injuries require immediate rest, cooling, compression, and elevation. The most important of these, cooling and compression, are denied to tissues encased in plaster.

Second, depending on the type of fracture, the soft tissues should receive regular massage after a short time.

Third, after the cast has been removed, the bone should not be highly stressed until increased massage pressures are tolerable.

These problems are rarely addressed, and the overall effect of conventional treatment is to produce a misshapen, rigid fracture site that is prone to frequent swelling. Fortunately, massage therapy – which includes hydrotherapy – is able to help the repair process, even if it is delayed until many years after the injury occurred.

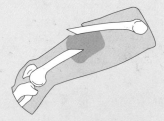

ATTENTION

The massage therapies described on the following pages were devised by a professional practitioner after informed assessment of the patients' injuries. In principle, there is no reason why massage given on an amateur basis should not be equally beneficial, but beware! If something goes wrong, causing further injury, the patient may be encouraged to sue for legal damages – which could be very expensive.

COMMON TYPES OF FRACTURE

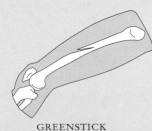

GREENSTICK

This is an incomplete fracture, rather like a broken sapling, which commonly occurs in a child or younger person.

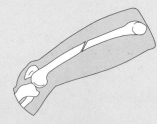

SIMPLE

The bone is partially or completely cracked but remains in reasonable alignment. Occasionally goes undiagnosed.

COMPOUND

Not only has the bone been broken and displaced but it pierces the skin. This increases dramatically blood loss.

CASE STUDY 5

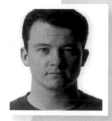

Name: Paul
Age: 33
Personal circumstances: Married, three children, manager of small printing works
Medical history: Enjoys good general health
Presenting: Wrist fracture: right-angle break to distal radius, plus longitudinal break to ulna
Referred by: Self

NOTES
• Active, athletic
• Qualified sports massage therapist

PAUL QUALIFIED AS a sports massage therapist and set up a meeting with his company's soccer team. Unfortunately, before he could impress them with his skills, he suffered a fractured wrist during a warmup session. The local casualty department confirmed that Paul had a double fracture and immediately encased his lower arm in a plaster cast. He was told he would need the cast for at least six weeks and that he should make small hand movements to prevent swelling.

PROBLEM	ASSESSMENT	TREATMENT
• Weight of cast causing stiffness • Some pain and swelling • Lack of faith in conventional therapy	• Plaster cast unnecessary • General health good • Fracture likely to respond to massage treatment	• STAGE 1: hydrotherapy • STAGE 2: cooling effleurage • STAGE 3: light petrissage

PAUL KNEW THAT fractures can be treated without resorting to plaster casts, so he consulted his massage teacher for advice. After some discussion he decided to try an alternative treatment.

STAGE ONE

The plaster cast was removed. Paul's hand was supported while cool water was poured repeatedly from the fingers to the elbow. This treatment was carried out twice a day for one week. Between treatments the arm was bandaged with cotton for protection, and a molded splint was inserted to keep the hand and arm in alignment.

STAGE TWO

During the second week, Paul continued to cool the arm as before, and applied gentle contact effleurage using cold soapy water. By week three he could perform the treatments with the lower arm upright to maximize drainage.

Feeling well, Paul visited the same hospital to attend an appointment three weeks after the fracture. The doctor did not seem particularly concerned about the disappearance of the plaster cast, and arranged to have the arm X-rayed again. A little later the doctor reassured Paul that the X-ray showed excellent healing for a five-week-old fracture, and suggested it would not need another week in plaster.

Paul could not resist reminding the doctor that his fracture was only three weeks old. Without further comment, the doctor redirected him to the plasterer.

Removing the new cast was easier than before, as Paul's arm was more comfortable. The cooling massage was resumed, and continued for two weeks.

STAGE THREE

During Paul's final hospital appointment the wrist was subjected to stress tests, and although these introduced pain for the first time since the fracture, the doctor concluded that the arm should be strongly exercised. This advice contradicted the massage treatment program, so light petrissage was applied instead, followed by cooling effleurage. Otherwise the arm was rested.

Over the next two weeks Paul visited a seawater pool twice daily, and he became able to use his arm for normal swimming. Three months after the fracture, Paul's wrist showed no noticeable signs of having been injured, and after five months he could perform one-arm push-ups.

CASTING OFF THE CAST

A plaster cast helps to align a fracture, but it postpones therapeutic activity. It is often better to replace the cast with splint bandages, or a lightweight polystyrene cast that can be undone to allow access for massage.

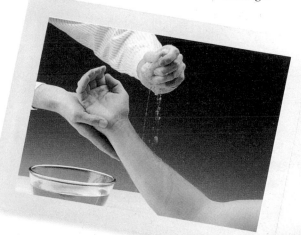

STAGE 1: HYDROTHERAPY

Cool-water hydrotherapy is ideal for an injury such as a fracture. It is most beneficial when applied as soon as possible, and for as long as necessary, after a trauma.

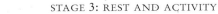

AVOID PAIN

Any rehabilitation exercises that cause pain are premature. Early movement does not prevent stiffness; it irritates the injury and actually makes stiffness more likely. Pain also leads to discomfort and deflates the patient's morale, and this in itself can impede recovery.

STAGE 3: REST AND ACTIVITY

Muscular fitness returns naturally to an injured area after more delicate structures have been repaired during complete rest, and there is freedom from pain. Only then will strengthening exercises prove beneficial.

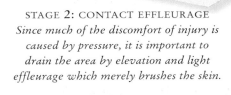

STAGE 2: CONTACT EFFLEURAGE

Since much of the discomfort of injury is caused by pressure, it is important to drain the area by elevation and light effleurage which merely brushes the skin.

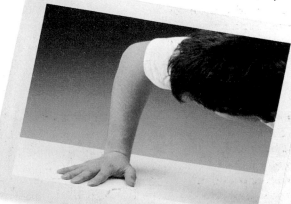

DAMAGED JOINTS

IF YOU WATCH the precision and flexibility of a dancer or gymnast, it is obvious that the body is capable of such actions because of the varied ways in which the human skeleton is joined together. The muscles may move the bones, but the accuracy with which we perform a multitude of tasks is achieved through the agency of the joints. Damage to the joints dramatically impairs movement, but massage can help restore their full function.

THERE ARE THREE major ways in which joints function. Before a baby is born, whole pieces of the skeleton, such as the skull, are loosely jointed. This allows the structure to collapse somewhat when passing through the birth canal. After birth, the pieces of bone in the skull become fused into a relatively solid whole.

In other places, such as the pelvis and chest, the bones never fuse. Instead, they are joined in a flexible fashion that allows movement but maintains firm support for the structures they contain or carry. These structures are relatively rigid, though, so most people do not recognize them as joints.

When we think of joints, we relate most directly to those in our arms and legs. We move these joints consciously, and the movement is very apparent. In these mobile joints the bones are freely articulated within a highly lubricated capsule, adapted to provide a high degree of flexibility.

In general, joints are very efficient, and have the capacity to remain problem-free throughout a lifetime's use. They can suffer, however, from the common disorder known as arthritis. This is sometimes considered a wear-and-tear condition, but there are respectable hypotheses to suggest that inflammatory conditions of the hands or feet involve significant emotional factors, such as resistance to certain tasks or aims. Massage is very helpful for someone who is aware of this type of conflict.

Although the joints are well protected from excessive movement by the ligaments, they are liable to dislocate if unexpectedly or inappropriately used. The most common example of this is where the arm is outstretched as protection from a fall, and transfers the impact to the shoulder. Sometimes the shock is absorbed by a fracture of the wrist or collar bone, but, if not, the head of the upper arm is apt to be jolted out of place. This requires immediate, possibly surgical intervention, but during the recovery period massage can help ensure a smooth, coordinated return to full functioning.

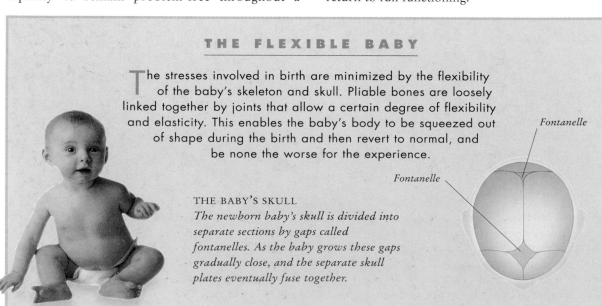

THE FLEXIBLE BABY

The stresses involved in birth are minimized by the flexibility of the baby's skeleton and skull. Pliable bones are loosely linked together by joints that allow a certain degree of flexibility and elasticity. This enables the baby's body to be squeezed out of shape during the birth and then revert to normal, and be none the worse for the experience.

Fontanelle

Fontanelle

THE BABY'S SKULL
The newborn baby's skull is divided into separate sections by gaps called fontanelles. As the baby grows these gaps gradually close, and the separate skull plates eventually fuse together.

HAND MASSAGE FOR ARTHRITIS

The heat generated by an inflamed joint does not respond favorably to direct massage. However, the surrounding areas appreciate drainage strokes since arthritis attracts lymphatic fluid, which helps to cool the joint and restrict movement. It is tempting to imagine that massage could free up an arthritic joint but in practice this would not happen. The joint's tension, after all, is controlled by muscles passing over it, so it is better to direct the massage to the non-inflamed parts of the muscles. External pressure may initially feel helpful due to counter-irritation, but the joint will react with increased inflammation soon afterward. If the patient feels like moving the joint gently after the draining massage, be encouraging. A little neutral massage oil, such as grapeseed, can be used to help deflect the pressure of the strokes.

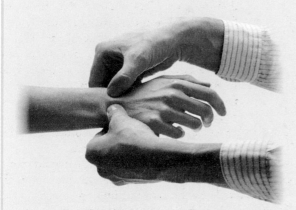

1 Do light effleurage of the hand and forearm. If the wrist joint is unaffected, petrissage all around and up into the forearm with fingertips and thumbs. Squeeze the wrist between the fingers and articulate the bones gently. Do firm effleurage up into the forearm. If the wrist is inflamed, effleurage only.

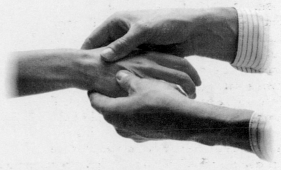

2 Effleurage the back of the hand, making fanning strokes with your thumbs from the knuckles to the wrist as if to spread the hand out. Then turn the hand over and, using the heel of your hand, effleurage the palm.

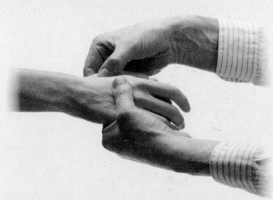

3 Turn the palm over. Using the edge of your thumb, petrissage the space between the thumb and first finger, up to the wrist and back, three times. Do firm effleurage in the space up to the wrist three times. Repeat in the spaces between the other bones of the hand.

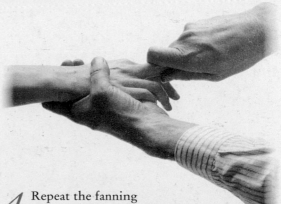

4 Repeat the fanning effleurage. Support the hand and gently wring the fingers, separating and straightening them, from knuckles to fingertips. Petrissage unaffected fingers by squeezing along the sides and pinching at the tips. Complete by effleuraging from fingertips to forearm, with hand raised, six times.

CASE STUDY 6

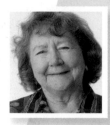

Name: Laurita
Age: 65
Personal circumstances: Widowed ex-social worker who lives alone
Medical history: Generally in good health, but finding that she tires easily
Presenting: Diagnosed osteoarthritis of hip joint, involving low back pain
Referred by: Medical doctor, after consultation for back pain
NOTES
• She likes to socialize, and particularly enjoys dancing

L AURITA DEVELOPED pain in her hip joint which progressed from intermittent to fairly constant. She became aware of decreased flexibility in her hip, and found that she was beginning to walk with a limp. An X-ray investigation suggested significant wear on the head of her femur, which, since it was accompanied by inflammation, painted a classic picture of osteoarthritis.

PROBLEM	ASSESSMENT	TREATMENT
• Osteoarthritis in the hip • Low back pain • Limping gait	• Back pain related to distortion of posture caused by hip problem • Affected leg noticeably shorter than the other • Poor mobility of affected leg	• Deep back massage to relieve tension • Deep leg massage and traction • Mobilization of the damaged hip joint

THE MEDICAL DIAGNOSIS of osteoarthritis did not in itself offer any relief for Laurita's hip, and on the advice of her doctor she resolved to take pain-killing drugs and to live with it. This is the only conventional therapy available for many musculo-skeletal disorders, but in the case of osteoarthritis of the hip there is an option: surgical replacement of the hip joint. This was available to Laurita, but at this point she felt that her back pain was a more urgent problem.

FIRST TREATMENT

Observation and tests showed that Laurita's backache was directly related to her postural accommodation of the arthritic hip. It is not uncommon for joint problems to disorganize the posture, particularly when they involve weight-bearing structures like the hips or knees. Inflammation can also affect nerves in nearby tissues and cause extended referred pain in distant parts of the body. Pain-killing drugs can make the problem worse, because although they mask the joint pain itself, they tend to cause strain in other areas by reducing sensitivity and encouraging over-use of the damaged tissues.

The tension in Laurita's back was dramatically reduced by general massage of the pelvic and spinal regions in the face-down position. Deep massage was not painful until the strokes penetrated the region of the affected hip. Laurita found that massage brought relief to her back and neck muscles.

When she turned over to face upward on the couch, Laurita found that her hip was still very painful, even after relaxing back massage. She could flex her knee only a little from the mid-line before experiencing pain. When she was lying full length, the affected leg appeared one inch shorter than the other.

TRACTION
During the first treatment session, the affected leg was massaged and given traction by pulling from the ankle.

The whole leg was massaged and given painless strong traction by pulling from the ankle until the leg lengths were approximately the same. Laurita was then shown how to apply gravitational traction at home by letting her affected leg extend from a stairway.

SECOND TREATMENT

On her second visit, Laurita said she had found the back massage helpful, and that her back pain was slightly improved. But her hip discomfort had apparently increased, even though she found that the stairway traction relieved some of the pressure on the joint.

The back massage was repeated, including the deep strokes to the postural muscles. The leg was then massaged, paying individual attention to the thigh muscles and performing general drainage effleurage of the buttocks.

Attempts to mobilize the hip using passive techniques were not helpful, since Laurita found

---

HOW DID MASSAGE HELP?

- The body devotes a lot of energy to pain management. The release of this energy through massage led to a surge of positive activity that may have brought forward the day when medical intervention was needed, but ultimately this may have been for the best.
- Massage can be very effective as a way of clarifying priorities, and this makes it a useful complementary therapy where surgery is inescapable.

---

it hard not to anticipate the movements. Resistive exercise – in which she used her knee to counter the pressure of the therapist's hand in different directions – proved much more successful, and led to increased flexibility of the hip joint.

Leg tractions, also from the knee, were effective in lengthening the leg and further reducing pressure in the affected hip joint.

FURTHER TREATMENTS

After this Laurita attended for treatment two or three times a week, and the results were both encouraging and disappointing. The massage helped to control

her problem with postural deviation from the hip, and the treatment reduced the inflammation in the damaged joint. Yet when she became tired, her hip pain recurred more intensely. Despite this the treatments were continued, and Laurita found that she gained considerable relief on the massage couch. There were occasions when the relief lasted for some considerable time after the massage therapy.

As the condition of her hip deteriorated, Laurita decided to face the inevitability of surgery, and subsequent treatments were oriented toward preparing her for the operation. The procedure was successful and she was able to use massage as part of her rehabilitation program.

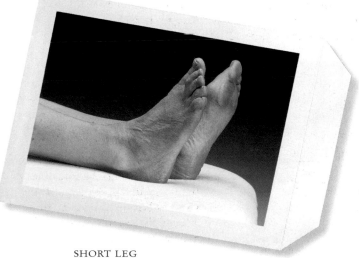

SHORT LEG
A hip problem can cause postural distortion that makes one leg look shorter than the other.

STAIRWAY TRACTION
Simply allowing the leg to extend from a stairway helps to counter the distortion and pain introduced by a damaged hip.

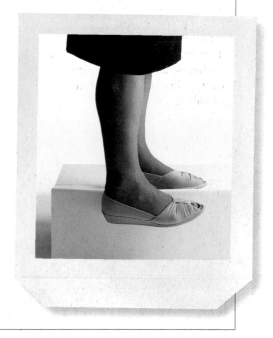

MASSAGE AND THE SPINE

IT SHOULD BE NO surprise that massage practitioners are frequently called upon to treat problems associated with the spine, for most people over the age of 45 years suffer low back or neck difficulties at some time. This is not to suggest, however, that spinal problems are inevitable, or that the spinal column is inherently weak.

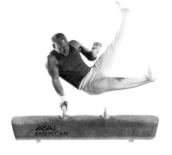

CONSIDERING THE adaptations that our posture has made to the modern world, it might be appropriate to review the "bad back" as the "back treated badly." In this light, the strain on the posture of a rural East African, denied the apparently helpful conveniences of modern technology, compares interestingly with that experienced by a typical Westerner.

In one study, researchers recorded stresses in the musculature of backpacking European tourists, and compared the results with similar measurements taken from Kenyan village women routinely carrying heavy containers of water on their heads. They found that whereas the backpackers' muscles became steadily more stressed and less efficient with increased loading, the villagers could support up to 20 percent of their body weight before recording any increase in muscle stress. Clearly the backpack is a far less efficient way of carrying heavy loads, and this inefficiency soon becomes evident as back pain.

Excessive muscular tension that causes back pain may also have emotional origins. In a recent practice experience, a slowly responding low back problem disappeared overnight to be replaced by incapacitating laryngitis – this on the morning of the patient's wedding day.

It is a common finding in massage therapy that treatment that reduces the inflammation near the spine is very helpful, even when the condition is described in terms of "bony displacement" or "trapped nerve." The counterirritation offered by massage is also useful when there is postural instability, such as exists around the time of menstruation. The unstable pelvis can increase pressure near the spinal nerves; this is referred to already congested abdominal vessels, which produces more pain. Massage reconstructs the advice, "Don't wash your hair during a period" to "Your period is making you vulnerable to low back pain caused by bending over."

TREATMENT

Corrective treatment to the spinal area involves a combination of massage, mobilization, and traction. Soothing and stimulating massage can relieve pain by reducing pressure and increasing the suppleness of the spine's muscles. On occasion, where the discs between the individual spinal bones have suffered serious degenerative changes, a qualified practitioner can be consulted for guidance. If massage is declined, this should be respected. It may be that the person's reservation about being touched is an intuition that the body is too busy with self-healing to be disturbed, even by massage.

Passive mobilization of the spine by gentle stretches aims to release tension around the joints, which are able to "give" slightly. Sometimes a "click" is heard on stretching, which often coincides with a sensation of relief. Although sometimes quite loud, the click is not a sign of overstretching, and no clinician has been able to give a convincing explanation for it.

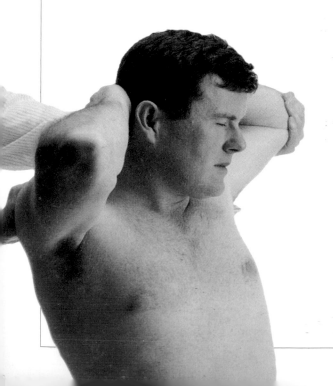

Traction is sometimes offered as a medical treatment under general anesthetic. While anesthesia is undeniably a form of relaxation, it is an illogical approach to spinal problems since the skeletal muscles, being voluntary, soon resume their former tension when consciousness returns. By contrast, the tractions of massage depend on the cooperative response of the patient, and help realign spinal posture after the acute discomfort is relieved.

Without very sophisticated equipment to detect minute circulatory and neurological changes in the body, you can never be quite sure that your corrections have been successful. Patients usually appreciate help, but may still complain of pain or stiffness after the treatment. Sometimes, in spite of their comments, it is easy to see that an improvement has taken place simply by the way they get dressed or describe their pain.

An indication of change can often be detected in the patient's facial expression. There is something about the quality of back and neck pain that is expressed in the face: if your patient looks relieved, smiles more, or engages you with their eye, you have probably helped a great deal.

COMMON SPINE PROBLEMS

TRAPPED NERVE
Nerves cannot actually become "trapped," but they can be pinched by misaligned vertebrae where they exit the spinal column. This usually occurs at the neck, causing tingling or numbness in the arm or fingertips.

LORDOSIS
The inward curve of the lumbar spine deepens in response to high heels, during pregnancy, and when the antagonistic abdominal muscles become unfit. The unrelieved pressure this creates will eventually provoke other spinal problems.

KYPHOSIS
The thoracic spine supporting the rib-cage can develop an exaggerated outward curve which distorts the shoulders and collapses the chest. This restricts breathing and puts pressure on the abdominal organs.

SCOLIOSIS
Uneven muscular development at the shoulders or pelvis can cause lateral deviations in the spinal column, creating a lateral "S" curve. The head may be tilted to compensate, to align the eyes with the horizon.

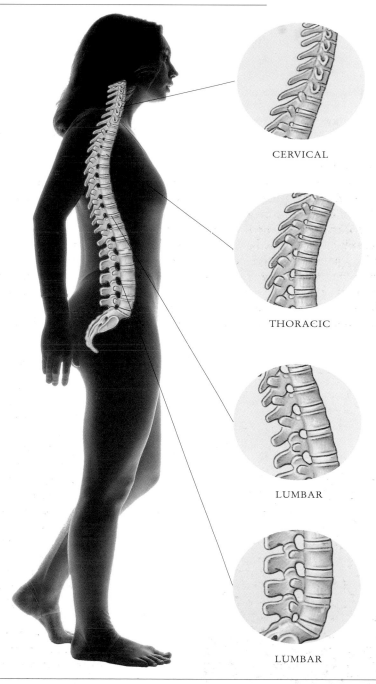

CERVICAL

THORACIC

LUMBAR

LUMBAR

Spinal Problems

THE MAJORITY OF back problems are caused by distortions of the spinal column's natural curvature. These can be caused by occupations that call for repeated actions involving one set of muscles, traumas arising from injury, or congenital conditions that have been compounded by the strains of adulthood. Either or all of these can lead to compensations in posture which give rise to inflammation and pain.

SPINAL PROBLEMS usually respond to a combination of massage and mobilization. The massage strokes increase circulation and relieve stiffness around the spine, while the gentle, rhythmic movements of mobilization encourage flexibility and strength.

The most common cause of spinal problems is lordosis, an inward curve of the lumbar spine. This part of the spine suffers from extremes of posture in everyday use, since it is often either braced bolt upright or collapsed in a slouch. It usually copes well, and any problems can often be traced to long periods of sitting, perhaps behind the driving wheel. The lumbar vertebrae are not supported by surrounding structures, such as the rib-cage above or the pelvis below, so they rely heavily on the

antagonistic muscles in the abdomen and waist. Consequently the most appropriate treatment is to loosen and "wring out" their increased tension as shown here, and give remedial exercises such as inverted postures, which avoid stressing the lumbars and improve the tone of the waist muscles. These movements are shown on pages 202–203.

The problem known as kyphosis tends to affect spinal posture with age, and is associated with the image of a an older, tired body. It is also an occupational disorder, however, which affects the increasing numbers of people who spend long hours at a desk. The thoracic vertebrae lose their ability to move, and this tends to strain the spine both below and above, particularly at the base of the neck.

MASSAGE TREATMENT FOR LORDOSIS

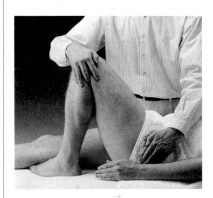

1 Flex the knee, placing the big toe under the opposite knee. Place the middle finger of your hand behind the knee.

2 Lever the patient's femur across toward you, while your other hand encourages the pelvis to rotate from the couch.

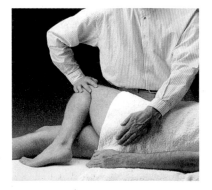

3 Steady the opposite shoulder and limit the rotation to a slight raising of the shoulder. Return the body to center, repeat the movements with the other leg, then mobilize the side that is more tense a second time.

After the freeing treatment described here, the thoracic spine should subjected to gentle traction, either by reaching up and holding firmly while the weight of the body is taken through the arms or, again, by inversion. This can be done by simply lying back, head downward on a incline, and raising the arms over the head. The inversion therapy technique is also an ideal treatment for kyphosis.

The lateral distortion known as scoliosis is more common than you might think. Since few people are naturally ambidextrous, there is a degree of scoliosis in everyone's spine. This tendency to favoritism is even present in the legs, since people usually select their strongest leg to begin the ascent of a flight of stairs. A psychological manifestation of scoliosis sometimes begins in childhood. Tensions representing conflicts of family loyalties are able to distort the developing musculature, and this affects the child's posture. For this reason all scoliosis treatments should include a review of family history.

The sequences shown here assume that a preparatory massage has taken place. Where the muscles are tender to the pressure of kneading, it is more appropriate to make friction strokes at right angles to the muscle fibers near the areas of pain. If the body "clicks" during a mobilization, this is a sign of helpful movement – but it is not necessary to "click the patient." The click is not made by bony or hard tissue, but by a release of pressure rather like removing the tongue from the roof of the mouth.

MASSAGE TREATMENT FOR KYPHOSIS

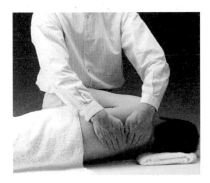

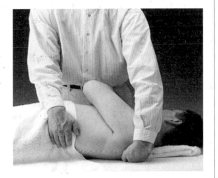

1 Stand close to the couch and reach over to place both hands under the shoulder, fingertips toward the spine. Bending your knees rhythmically, rotate the upper body from the couch.

2 Continuing to rotate, gradually move the lower hand down the far side of the back, alternately rotating with the upper hand then the lower hand to wriggle the body. When your hand reaches the pelvis, place it carefully on the outer rim.

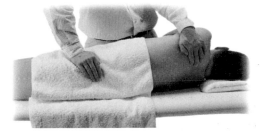

3 Make one final rotation of the upper body, with the patient breathing out, as you fix the pelvis and slowly draw the shoulder as much as possible from the couch. Repeat to the other side, then again to the more restricted side.

MASSAGE TREATMENT FOR SCOLIOSIS

1 Have the patient sit on the couch with his hands lightly clasped behind his head. Place your right hand in front of his right elbow and your palm against his left scapula. On an outbreath, rotate the patient to the right, gently pulling on the elbow, steadying the body at the scapula. Hold at a comfortable limit. On a further outbreath, increase the stretch and hold for three seconds. Return the body smoothly to center and repeat to other side. Mobilize the tighter side a second time.

CASE STUDY 7

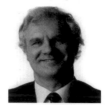

Name: Christopher
Age: 60
Personal circumstances: Single; professor of history
Medical history: History of mild back spasm
Presenting: Acute spasm in lower back
Referred by: Self

NOTES
• Keeps fit by gym training and through swimming

CHRISTOPHER CONTACTED his massage therapist from home. He had been getting out of his car when his back seized up and he had only just managed to walk to the house. He was unable to stand upright and had radiating pains along the back of one leg, extending to the sole of his foot. His massage practitioner arranged to visit Christopher at home, and meanwhile advised him to immobilize his back by lying on his side with his knees drawn up and a pillow between them. He was advised against taking painkillers.

SYMPTOMS	ASSESSMENT	TREATMENT
• Spasm in back	• Spinal deviation	• Immobilization as first
• Inability to stand up	• Twisted pelvis	aid
• Radiating pain in	• Raised shoulders	• Back and abdominal
one leg		massage
		• Rehabilitation
		exercises

FIRST TREATMENT

When the therapist visited him later that day, Christopher was still having problems standing, but the pain in his leg was much less severe.

Examination of his back in the upright position showed spinal deviation and twisting of the pelvis. Christopher slowly dropped on to his hands and knees and was gradually placed face down on the floor with a large bed pillow under his abdomen. He was given gentle massage of the whole back, with warming effleurage strokes and frictions. As the treatment progressed, Christopher was able to relax over the pillow and began to feel the spasm in his back releasing.

Christopher turned over, keeping his knees flexed, until he was lying flat with his feet close to his buttocks. The therapist then administered gentle swaying movements to his thighs so that his pelvis rocked lightly to the left and right. This helped stretch the back muscles and unwind the pelvic rotation.

Christopher then resumed a position on hands and knees, and while the therapist supported his arms he was slowly helped to first kneel upright, then stand up, one leg at a time. He was then instructed to retract his abdominal muscles firmly, let go of the therapist, and confidently walk around the room. He achieved this, and felt much relief. He was advised to take short, hot baths if pain returned, and to rest with the pillow between his legs as before.

SECOND TREATMENT

Two days later Christopher was able to make his way to the treatment clinic. He was in less pain, although he still showed spinal deviation with a twisted pelvis and raised shoulders.

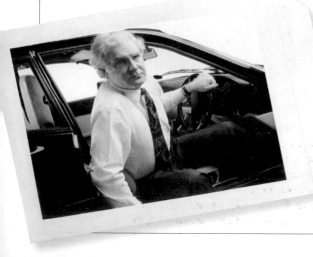

RISK POSTURE
The most common cause of back muscle spasm is bending sideways while in rotation, as when attempting to get out of a car with one leg supporting the weight of the body. This posture puts intense pressure on the spinal joints and invariably results in a protective but painful spasm of the back muscles.

He received back and abdominal massage using slow, deep kneading and draining effleurage. The massage strokes felt welcome and Christopher felt the muscles in his back let go. To his surprise he suddenly experienced deep exhaustion and his head began to swim. The therapist was aware of his disorientation and quietly reassured him that any strange sensations were a result of his muscles returning to their normal tone. The session was completed with deep breathing exercises which helped Christopher integrate the effects of the treatment.

He was then instructed in daily rehabilitation exercises to aid recovery. These consisted of gentle twisting stretches to release muscle cramping, and single leg squatting with one foot stepped up on a table to help realign the spinal posture. He was warned against strenuous movements, especially with the legs kept straight, but encouraged to take up normal activity.

SEEK PROFESSIONAL ADVICE

If untutored massage increases back pain, seek professional help as soon as possible. Back pain is rarely caused by one event; it usually reflects a build-up of pressure around the spinal joints over a period of time. Professional attention has an impressive reputation for treating back problems, not least in providing important support to deal with the loss of confidence experienced by many back sufferers.

THIRD TREATMENT

Christopher returned for a conditioning massage and to have his exercise programme reviewed after two weeks, and reported that he was feeling fitter and more energetic than before his acute back spasm.

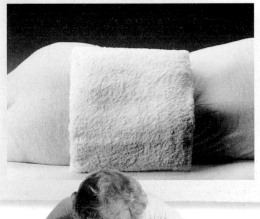

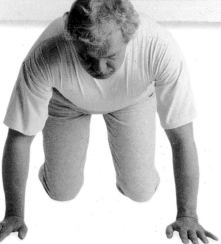

SELF-HELP: HOT COMPRESS
If massage is not available for acute spasm, try a hot compress or hot bath. The treatment should be of short duration, lasting up to 10 minutes, or the muscles will tend to become overcooked and will get more painful.

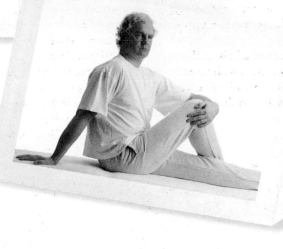

KNEELING ON ALL FOURS
The instinctive response to back muscle spasm is to lean forward onto the hands, and ultimately kneel on all fours. This is ideal since it decreases pressure on the spine and can successfully release the spasm.

SELF-HELP: GENTLE EXERCISE
Experience indicates that coordination exercises combined with modest strengthening movements are beneficial during recovery from back pain. Yoga-derived positions, combined with deep breathing, flowing Tai Chi sequences, and gentle gymnastics are preferable to hyperextensions (raising the body from the floor) or punishing "sit ups."

MUSCLE AND TENDON INJURIES

PERHAPS MORE THAN any other system of the body, it is the muscles that are most popularly associated with massage therapy. This may be because massage has been traditionally used by all great movers – athletes, acrobats, dancers, and wrestlers. Muscles are extremely elastic, fibrous tissues. The skeletal muscles are striped, while the muscles of the internal organs have fibers that are relatively smooth. Their purpose is to pull us around in slightly different ways, as their appearance suggests: the former work rather suddenly, while the latter work in an altogether more restrained but equally determined way.

SKELETAL MUSCLE AND smooth muscle are also neurologically distinct. The muscles that move bones receive their nervous impulses consciously from the brain, so their actions are essentially voluntary. The muscles in the organs, by contrast, are moved by signals that we do not consciously control, so their actions are involuntary. Perhaps this is good, since it allows us to follow our interests in the outside world without neglecting our internal organs.

Sociable eating is a good example of how the two types of muscles function and, when necessary, communicate. Providing we render our meal fit to be swallowed by chewing it adequately, we can hold an intense conversation without being distracted by the fate of our food. If, as sometimes happens, the work of the mouth is incomplete, the food is unceremoniously regurgitated by the smooth muscle lining the esophagus, to receive further conscious attention. Generally speaking, the involuntary muscles have the greater power to override the voluntary muscles, and certainly have no regard for social etiquette.

INJURY AND DISORDER

Muscles renew and replenish themselves on a daily basis and will grow according to the demands placed upon them. When we are awake, the muscles are keen competitors for blood and will concentrate the circulation in areas where the greatest work is being done. If the organ muscles are competing for blood in this way, they will always attract the greater supply. If at such times the voluntary muscles are asked to perform an action without an adequate blood supply, they are at risk of strain or injury.

Muscular disorders are very common, and the constitution of muscles makes any injury debilitating and painful. Without appropriate treatment, skeletal muscles can become chronically dysfunctional, leading to further strain and immobility. The organ muscles become injured primarily through nervous

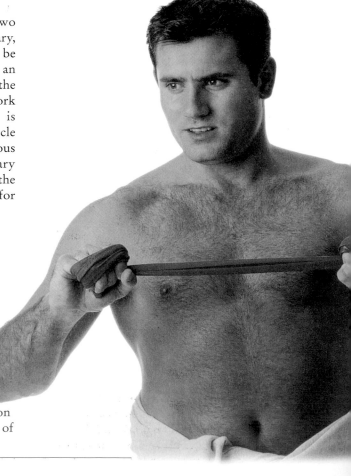

disorder, which produces an inflexibility in the major body systems. Cardiovascular complications are among the most well known of these conditions.

HOW MASSAGE CAN HELP

Massage is able to work directly with muscles because the practitioner's hands are themselves being moved by muscles, something to which the patient's brain is immediately alert. Before manipulation can begin, however, the treatment is always preceded by cooling hydrotherapy to contain swelling and inflammation, and ease pain. Chronic conditions respond well to contrasting hot and cold hydrotherapy, which has the effect of regressing an injury and revealing concealed problems.

TREATMENT

Treatment always begins with an assessment of mobility, since all injuries will involve a degree of compensation in nearby structures. This may involve a general body massage, distant from the site of injury or at the nearest spinal segment, which reveals the true extent of the injury. Direct pressure over the injury should only be given using contrasting hot and cold hydrotherapy.

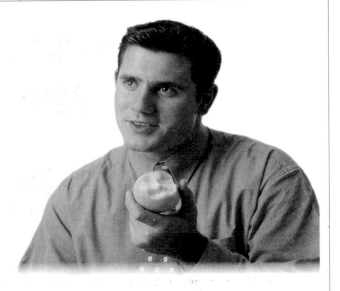

INVOLUNTARY MUSCLES
The internal musculature such as the digestive tract is not under conscious control. It may go into spasm but this is usually generated by nervous tension rather than overuse and is resolved by emotional rest.

When passive movement produces no pain, after-massage mobilization can be added to the treatment. The passive, active and resistive nature of these movements reeducate the injured area by stretching, strengthening and encouraging coordination.

The time taken for an injury to recover depends as much on the state of an injured person as the damage to the tissues involved. Provided rest is assured and the patient develops a calm but positive attitude, with the support of appropriate therapy, the body can release its enormous capacity for self-regeneration.

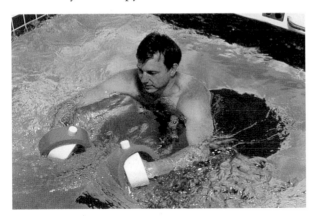

HYDROTHERAPY
Movements done underwater are more effective than other forms of exercise, because the body is always supported. Also, the muscles are in effect retraining themselves in a stimulating "reverse action."

MUSCLE TONE
Freely using our muscles keeps them comfortably tense, a condition known as "tone" but overuse can be as damaging as underuse. Many sportspeople find the relaxing effects of massage useful in maintaining fitness.

SPORTS INJURIES

While it may be impossible to avoid predictable sports injury completely, the most troublesome injuries are not from unexpected disaster but from overuse. This may occur, for example, when an attempt is made to play on although injured, or by returning to action before adequate healing has taken place. Regular massage will help maintain some degree of fitness while injured structures are healing.

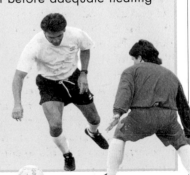

CASE STUDY 8

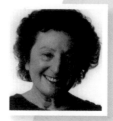

JAYNE HAD DAMAGED her shoulder three months before the first appointment, when turning from the driving seat of her car to retrieve a heavy briefcase from the seat behind. She had received physiotherapy with massage and ultrasound, and was given a sheet of exercises to perform. She found the massage painful and was unable to do the exercises.

Name: Jayne
Age: 49
Personal circumstances: Single; schoolteacher
Medical history: Has had neck problems after whiplash three years previously
Presenting: Painful shoulder, locked elbow
Referred by: Patient's Tai chi teacher, who was concerned about the deteriorating condition of her arm

NOTES
• Patient dedicated to her job
• Feels strained by conditions at work

SYMPTOMS	ASSESSMENT	TREATMENT
• Pain in shoulder • Stiffening elbow • Stiff neck	• Muscle tension in arm • Inflammation in shoulder • Reduced strength and mobility	• Massage • Contrast hydrotherapy • Mobilizing treatments

Although Jayne found the physiotherapy painful, she continued attending in the hope that the intensity of treatment would help her shoulder. In fact, the pain increased and, finding that her elbow was stiffening up, she abandoned the treatment. At this point she was recommended for massage therapy.

FIRST TREATMENT

Jayne's arm was found to be very tense. She was unable to raise her arm above shoulder level or straighten her elbow. There was inflammation around the shoulder, and her elbow was in spasm. She had reduced strength in her hand grip and was unable to turn her head satisfactorily.

Massage was first given to her neck muscles to help relieve the pressure on the spinal nerves leading down into the arm. The arm was effleuraged, and gentle wringing strokes applied to improve the circulation. A seated back massage addressed the tension that had built up in Jayne's posture. She was instructed to do contrast hydrotherapy using alternate hot and cold towels every other day for a week, and told to keep the arm rested.

SECOND TREATMENT

Jayne's arm was much more comfortable, and she had been able to sleep better at night. Muscle strength was improved, although she still had restricted mobility. Massage was repeated to her neck, including slow stretching. Her arm was treated with frictions at right angles to the muscle fibers, and deep draining effleurage was given. The elbow was moved passively, actively, and with resistance – movements that help to re-educate joints. She was instructed to continue the contrast hydrotherapy at home for two weeks.

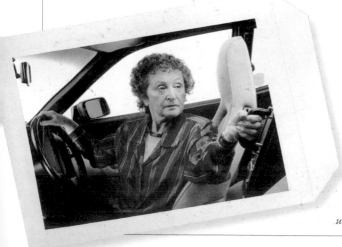

VULNERABLE MUSCLES
Shoulder or arm injuries usually involve the neck muscles. Jayne's attempt to lift a heavy briefcase from the back seat of her car is a typical cause of such damage, and anyone who has a previous history of neck problems is particularly vulnerable to this type of injury. Shoulder problems sometimes involve complications, and because of this they usually take a long time to recover fully.

THIRD TREATMENT

Jayne reported that her arm felt as if it now belonged to the rest of her body and demonstrated its improved flexibility. The friction massages on the neck and arm were repeated, and then the reeducation exercises were extended to include the shoulder. At the end of treatment both arm and shoulder showed increased flexibility. Jayne was instructed to reduce the hydrotherapy to twice weekly, and cautioned not to use her arm too enthusiastically.

FOURTH TREATMENT

After a month Jayne's confidence in her arm was returning and, with the exception of her shoulder, she was using it almost normally. She was given whole back and arm massage, and petrissage and kneading movements were used on the arm for the first time. She was also given coordination exercises that involved the back and arms. At the end of the treatment Jayne was able to clap her hands with her arms straight just above shoulder level.

After this Jayne attended four more monthly treatments and was able to clap her hands directly above her head at the beginning of the final treatment.

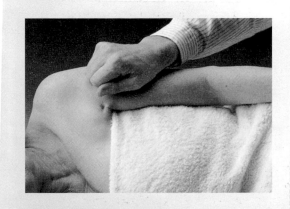

CONTRAST HYDROTHERAPY
Pressure massage strokes and exercises are not appropriate during the acute stage of muscle injury. The repairing capillaries are fragile and can be easily broken again, which leads to blood loss and bruising. Contrast hydrotherapy, using six alternate 30-second applications of hot and cold towels, is a safe, effective pain-relieving treatment.

FRICTION STROKES
Muscle injuries should be frictioned, and never kneaded or given petrissage. Friction strokes encourage drainage of the toxins that build up at the injury site, and encourage muscle regrowth. Muscle-building exercises only irritate the healing processes.

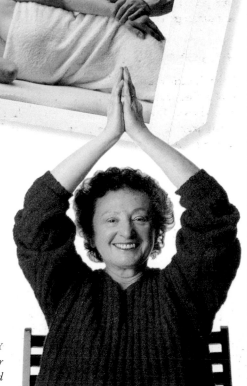

RECOVERY
By the end of her treatment. Jayne was able to clap her hands above her head – something that she had previously found unthinkable.

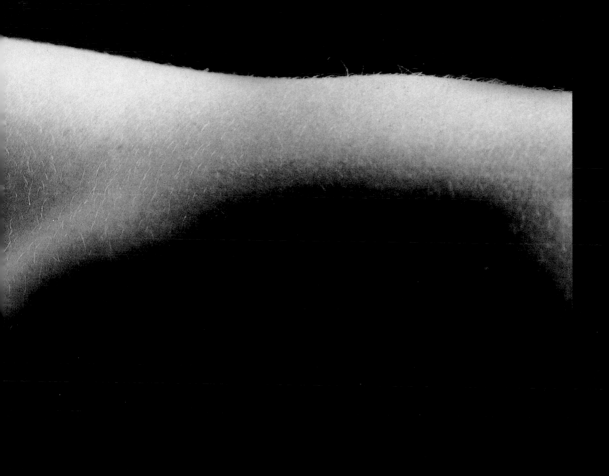

PART SEVEN

MASSAGE AS SELF-TREATMENT

While massage is generally most beneficial when given by another person, it can also be used as a safe and effective self-treatment. Practitioners often teach self-applied movements to use at home to extend the effects of a professional massage. There may also be occasions when treatment is required urgently, and such emergencies nearly always occur when helpful friends or therapists are unavailable. When the immediate need is to contain a problem or deal with acute pain, self-treatments can be extremely valuable. Quite apart from any physical benefit, the feeling that you are able to respond physically to a problem can be very reassuring as you await the attention of an expert therapist.

SELF-MASSAGE HAS a variety of applications. Chronic conditions and problems associated with wear and tear often respond well to self-treatment. It is very comforting to have techniques readily available that are helpful in managing pain, refreshing, and emotionally sustaining. Respiratory distress and exhaustion are two instances where self-massage is known to be beneficial. Self-massage can also provide stress relief in the workplace. In parts of China, for example, it is a recognized part of the daily routine of many workers. Occupationally, the most obvious practitioners of self-massage are massage therapists, who enjoy its benefits through the rhythmic strokes and movements they apply to their patients.

SELF-MASSAGE
You can apply self-massage whenever you need it, without delay.

A SOFTER OPTION

While self-treatment is primarily a maintenance therapy, it has a role in the prevention of problems. By including self-massage as part of a fitness program it is possible to avoid the build-up of conditions that may precede an emergency. Learning self-massage can also be an important step towards accepting treatment from someone else. If given massage feels too pressurizing or threatening for those who are reclaiming their bodies from self-harm or other type of trauma, tentative self-massage can encourage recognition of positive sensory experiences.

This is particularly true of reservations about abdominal massage. It is understandable that we should feel physically protective of the abdomen since, considering its importance, it is a relatively unprotected area of the body. It is quite possible that, because of the ideal position of our hands relative to the abdomen and the sensitivity of its muscles, self-massage of the abdomen may initially be more effective than given massage. The realization of its benefits may then allow a deeper, therapeutic treatment to be received from an experienced massager later.

SELF-MASSAGE IN PRACTICE

Given reasonable privacy, self-treatment can be applied wherever and whenever possible. There are some simple movements that can be done anywhere, such as squeezing the fists while walking or wriggling the toes within shoes; both of these are useful for relieving tiredness. It is also possible to apply self-help therapy at unreasonable or antisocial times, such as in the middle of the night. Self-applied neck massage, for example, can help deal with broken sleep.

Self-treatment is rarely contraindicated, even when given massage may be inadvisable. This is because you have total control over the level of pressure – an important feature of appropriate massage. There is also less chance that the treatment may irritate underlying conditions, because the feedback is immediate and the movements can be finely adjusted. Self-massage can even assist in reclaiming self-control after the disablement of illness or injury.

Applied massage treatment is more successful, of course, when self-control needs to be surrendered to the practitioner's hands. Self-massage can, therefore, only be taken so far as an emotional therapy. This is not to say that self-treatment cannot feel soothing or calming, merely that it does not deliver the helpful detachment and altered perspective provided by the experience of being massaged.

RELAXING YOUR SPINE

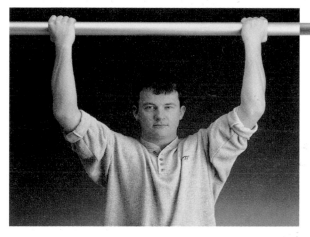

1 Find a doorway with a surround deep enough to allow you to comfortably reach up and hold on. Sports shops sell a telescopic handhold that can be adjusted to fit a door space.

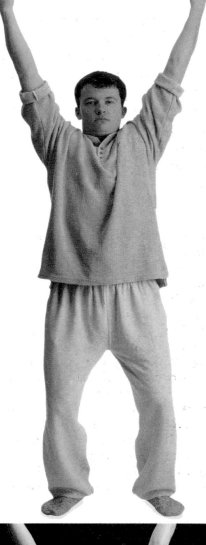

2 Breathe out and bend your knees slowly as if to sit on a stool. You will feel the muscles of the trunk lengthening, and pressure in the lower back will traction out. Hold for a few seconds at full stretch.

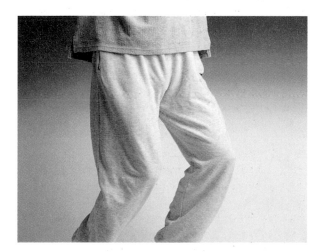

3 Draw your abdomen in firmly and slowly stand up, taking your weight on your feet again. Repeat as necessary. Stretching can be increased by rotating the lower half of the body on the balls of the feet in a gentle rhythm.

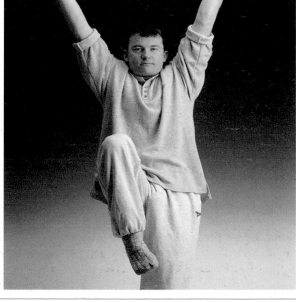

4 If you are aware of more tension to one side of your body, raise your knees alternately as high as possible, twice as much on the easier side.

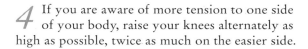

SELF-MASSAGE: BACK

Back PROBLEMS are so common that most people have experienced an occasion when their back apparently "goes." There is usually a split-second awareness of something not quite right in posture, followed by a seizing of all the muscles in the vicinity, if not the whole body. Although essentially a defensive reaction to safeguard the spine, the dramatic rise in muscular tension can result in a mild case of shock. The following sequence is recommended for spasm involving the lower back muscles. Rehearse the sequence now if you have a recurring back problem.

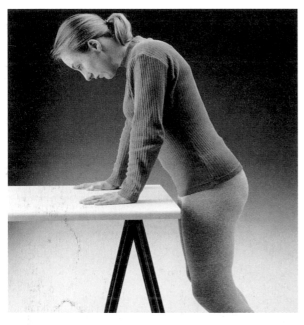

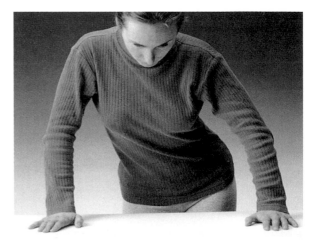

2 Breathe deeply to help relieve shock. It is likely that one side of the back is primarily affected and contracting nearby muscles for support, so detect which side is contracted most by moving your pelvis gently to left and right.

1 As soon as possible after the spasm, transfer some of the weight of your body from your legs to your arms by pressing on a nearby surface. If a spasm occurs when seated, go straight to position 4.

3 Slowly get down on all fours. Extend the leg on the tense side of your back and lower the rest of your body gently to the floor.

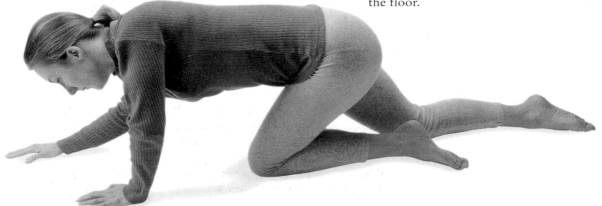

4 Draw the opposite knee toward your chest. Place your arm alongside and turn your head to face the same way.

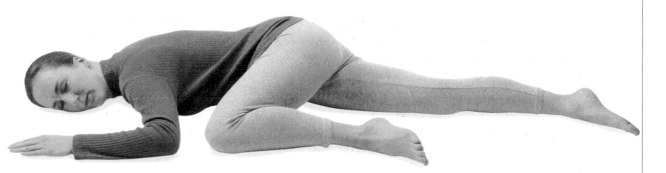

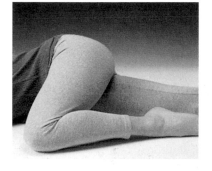

5 Rest, helping to release your back muscles further by firmly retracting your abdomen and imagining your body being compressed by the force of gravity.

6 When you are feeling calmer, return to the all-fours position and rest again. Slowly straighten up from kneeling by climbing up a piece of furniture. If another spasm occurs, return to the former position for a few more minutes.

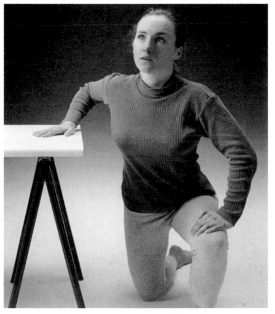

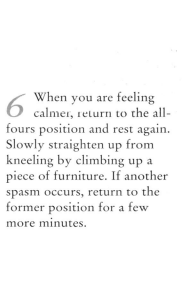

7 Climb up, one leg at a time, and stand erect with knees slightly bent. Hold your abdominal muscles as tight as possible. Don't feel defeated if you still have some pain. Your back will have improved more than you realize.

SELF-MASSAGE: NECK

THE NECK IS a vulnerable structure. The heels of shoes cause the head to tilt backwards and shorten the neck; most of us hear better from one ear and twist the neck around to the clearer side; violent movements may tear at the neck's delicate nerves and blood vessels. This in turn may lead to referred pains in the head and arms. Compensatory tensions build up around the bones, often heard as crackling during neck exercises. This self-massage encourages a relaxed centeredness of the neck. It is also worth trying for sinus congestion, with the addition of a hot cloth over the cheeks, and a cold cloth around the feet.

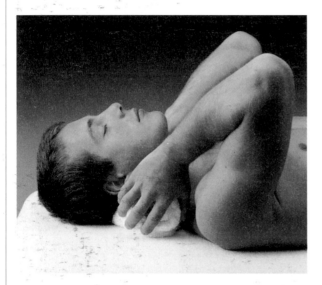

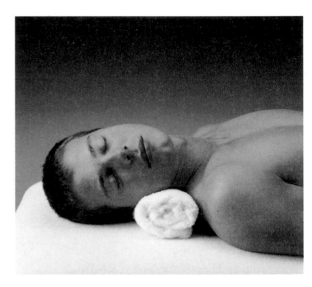

1 Roll a small towel to a diameter of roughly three inches. Lie down and place the towel directly beneath your neck, taking up the normal neck curvature. Relax your jaw.

3 Keeping your head in contact with the floor, roll to the left and right against the towel a few times, then come to rest on the right side. Breathe deeply for a few seconds.

2 Draw your feet up closer to your hips. Without deliberately moving, your head will have rocked slightly backward.

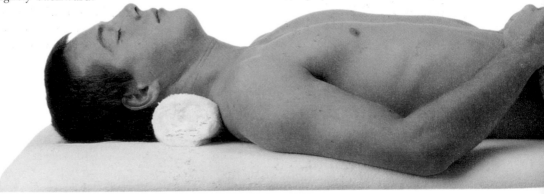

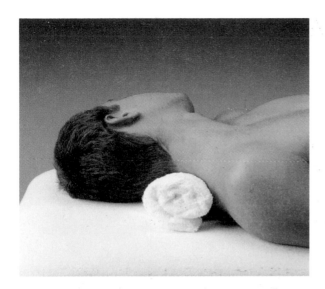

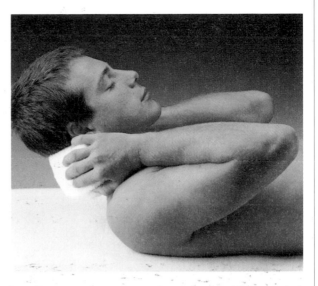

4 Roll again two or three times and rest on the left side, breathing as before. If one side of the neck feels tighter, roll the head back toward the stiffness for a few seconds, then slowly roll as far as possible in the opposite direction.

5 Return to center, reach up, and hold the ends of the towel. After a deep inward breath, exhale while at the same time rolling your supported head comfortably forward, chin toward your chest. Repeat once more.

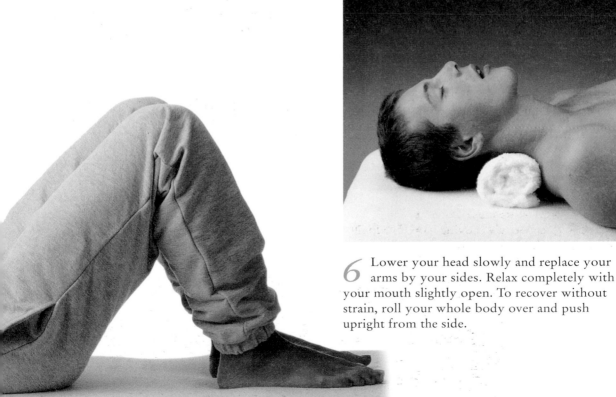

6 Lower your head slowly and replace your arms by your sides. Relax completely with your mouth slightly open. To recover without strain, roll your whole body over and push upright from the side.

SELF-MASSAGE: ABDOMEN

THE USUAL CAUSE of abdominal pain is indigestion. Excessive consumption of any food tends to overwhelm the system, and when someone is exhausted or nervously upset, food eaten is hardly processed at all. The pain associated with the symptoms is connected to the slow but steady cramping of the muscles of digestion, which normally squeeze food gently through the system. Since this process is itself a massage system for food, self-massage is a very appropriate treatment.

1 Lie down with a pillow under your knees. Take a few deep breaths. Investigate your abdomen with gently probing fingers. If you feel a tightening over a painful area, begin a smooth, continuous, reinforced effleurage, clockwise, and lighter over the uncomfortable part.

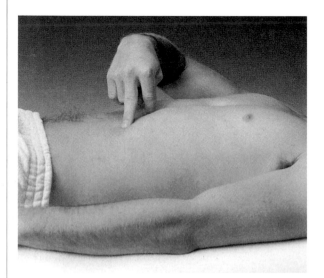

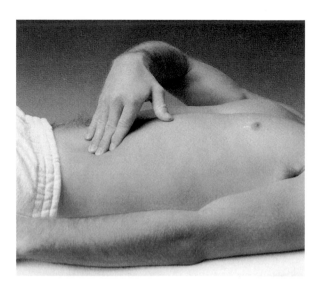

2 If this helps, use the knuckles or fingertips to give little bounces over the painful part, pressing enough to stretch the skin. You may detect some movement within the abdomen. Alternate this pressure with effleurage.

3 Where there has been focused tension in the abdomen, the remaining area will have gone slack. Do a quicker, upward effleurage with one or both hands to encourage toning.

SELF-MASSAGE: CONSTIPATION

THE INTERNAL BODY massage responsible for moving food through the digestive tract is called peristalsis. The action of peristalsis is continuous to the very end of the digestive process in the large intestine or colon, but action of the sympathetic nervous system can disrupt the activity of the colon and cause constipation. Self-massage can help relieve the problem by converting the sympathetic nervous activity to parasympathetic activity. The position adopted for this massage is well known outside English-speaking countries.

1 Practice squatting by holding on to a stable chair or door handle and lowering your hips between your feet. Try to keep your feet flat.

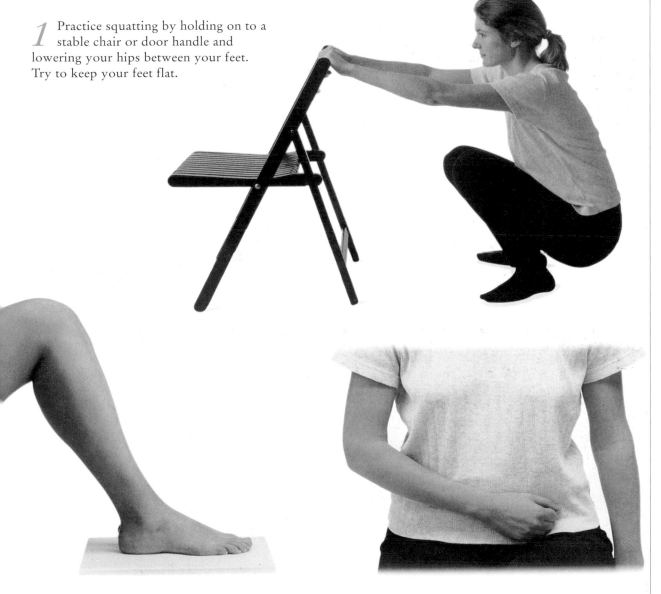

2 When you have made your hips supple, squat on the toilet seat in the same way. If you can't manage this without fear of falling, sit down and raise your feet on a box so that your knees are higher than your hips.

3 Retract and slowly release your abdomen a few times. Make a fist and press gently but deeply around the edge of the abdomen, especially on the left side. Relax and breathe deeply, and avoid bearing down.

SELF-MASSAGE: CIRCULATION

The CARDIOVASCULAR SYSTEM, which circulates blood through the body, relies on a degree of muscular activity to work effectively. Older people often find ways of economizing on such movements, and this tendency to slow down inevitably results in poorer circulation. Massage can be a valuable corrective therapy for this problem, and self-massage is both highly recommended and easy to achieve. The following techniques treat the chest by reflex action from the upper arms.

1 Place a folded towel behind your back at the level of the upper arms. Take up the slack against the skin and lean back slightly, hands not too far apart. Draw the towel to the right by extending your elbow, aiming to friction the arms.

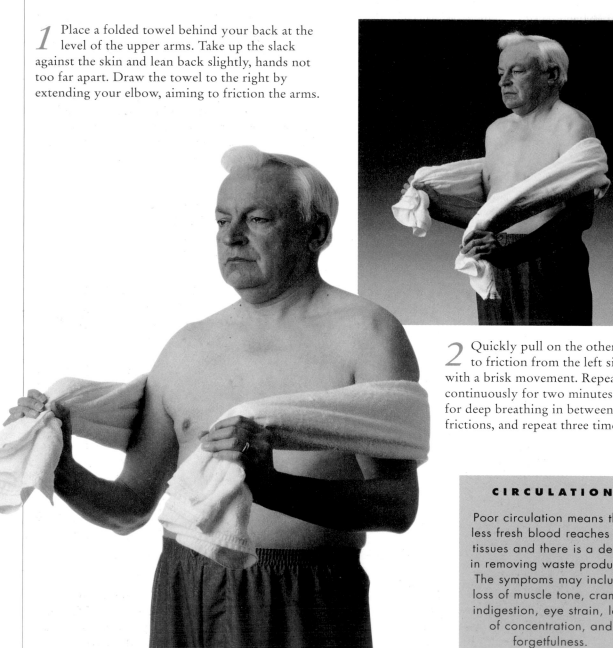

2 Quickly pull on the other hand to friction from the left side with a brisk movement. Repeat continuously for two minutes. Rest for deep breathing in between frictions, and repeat three times.

CIRCULATION

Poor circulation means that less fresh blood reaches the tissues and there is a delay in removing waste products. The symptoms may include loss of muscle tone, cramp, indigestion, eye strain, loss of concentration, and forgetfulness.

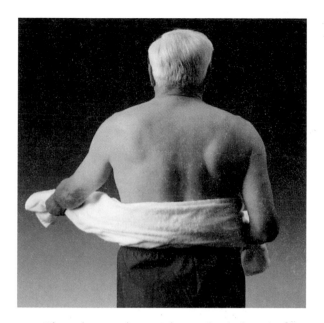

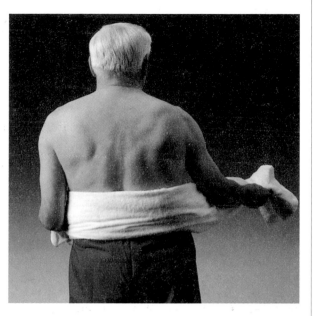

3 Place the towel around your back, keeping it tight, a little higher than the waist. Lean back slightly and give a vigorous pull to the left side, aiming to friction around the shape of the back.

4 Give an equally vigorous tug to the other side. Get a strong rhythm going and repeat until your back feels very warm. You can achieve a fuller back stroke by raising your elbows, but the focus should return to your kidney area.

5 Fold the towel and place it around your neck like a scarf. Lean your head back slightly, feeling the support from the towel. Draw the towel to the right with enough pressure on the neck to create a gentle friction.

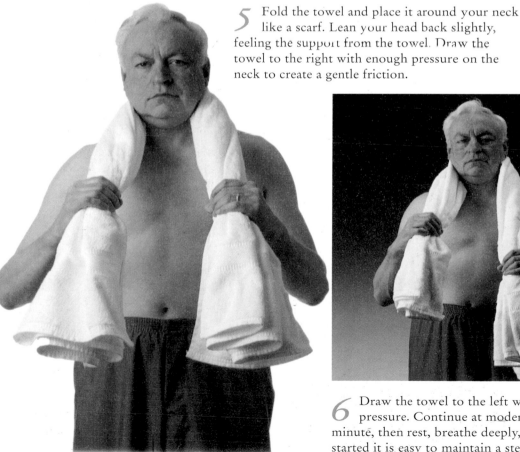

6 Draw the towel to the left with the same pressure. Continue at moderate speed for one minute, then rest, breathe deeply, and repeat. Once started it is easy to maintain a steady rhythm, but avoid intense friction.

SELF-MASSAGE: MENSTRUAL PAIN

THE DISCOMFORT EXPERIENCED during menstruation and after birth can be relieved by simply inverting the pelvis. This reduces pressure within the blood vessels and gives a welcome traction to the lower back. This self-treatment can be used to relieve discomfort as necessary, but may bring a long-term improvement if it is practiced throughout the cycle. Immediately after birth, begin the treatment by raising the legs at the lower end of the bed by three inches, and gradually progress to the full sequence.

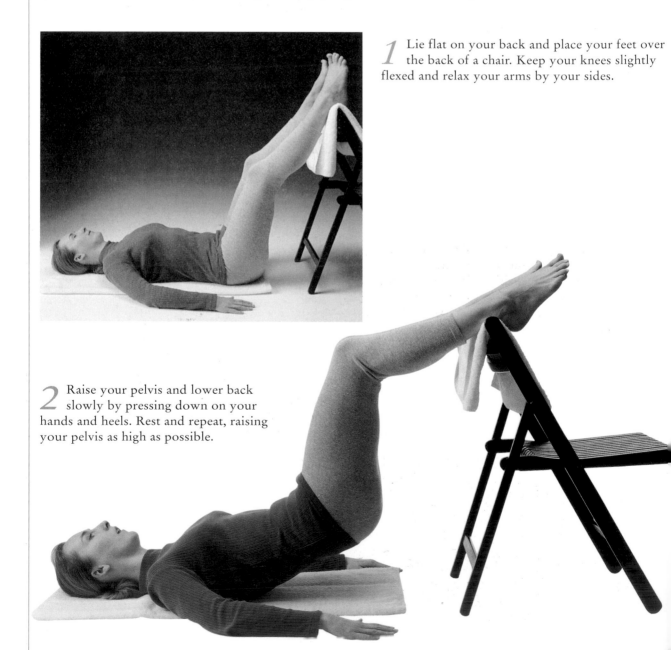

1 Lie flat on your back and place your feet over the back of a chair. Keep your knees slightly flexed and relax your arms by your sides.

2 Raise your pelvis and lower back slowly by pressing down on your hands and heels. Rest and repeat, raising your pelvis as high as possible.

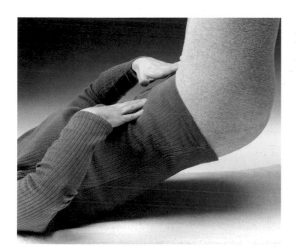

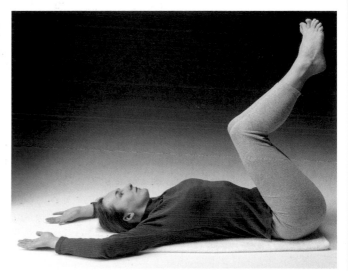

3 While your pelvis is raised, tense your legs to hold the position and gently scoop the abdomen from pelvis to rib-cage, with alternate hands. Lower slowly and do a simple effleurage of your abdomen and the tops of your thighs.

4 Place both arms over your head and breathe deeply. Draw your knees to your chest, keeping your back flat. Briefly drop your toes to the floor, then swing your legs into the air, rolling your pelvis and lower back up as high as possible.

5 Initially, your legs will tend to point beyond your head, but with practice you will achieve a more upright position. The point of this section of the treatment is to encourage a gentle struggle to remain in the air, so don't overstrain. Remain in the air for as long as you feel comfortable.

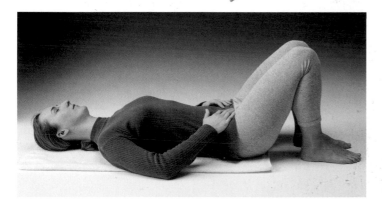

6 Recover by rolling down carefully on to your spine and pelvis. Place your feet close to your hips and rest for a while, breathing deeply.

SELF-MASSAGE: EYES

ALTHOUGH IT MAY not seem possible to overuse the eyes, the monotonous gazing and fixed focusing associated with modern living can become strenuous. The strain affects the eyes' external muscles, causing them to sting and ache. Eyesight is also known to be affected by stressful events. This self-massage, known as palming, has both physical and mental benefits. It deeply relaxes the eyes and eases tension in the neck muscles, which is important for the circulation to the eyes. If you are becoming concerned about your eyes, do these movements twice a day and seek neck massage.

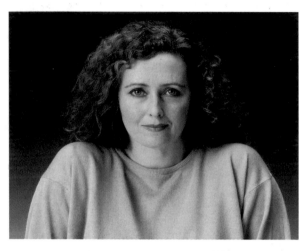

1 Wearing loose-necked clothing, sit close to a table. Shrug your shoulders, rolling forward and backward six times.

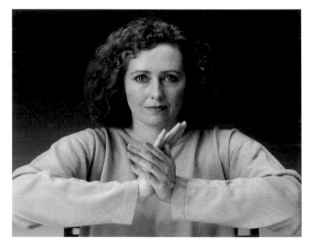

2 Rub your hands together vigorously for a few seconds to generate some friction and make them feel warm.

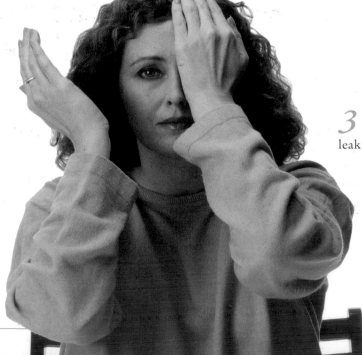

3 Place both your palms (not your fingers) over your closed eyes so that no light can leak through the gaps.

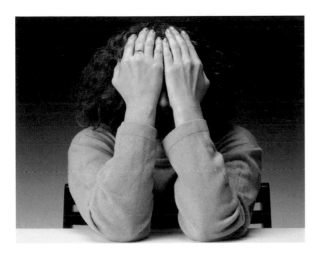

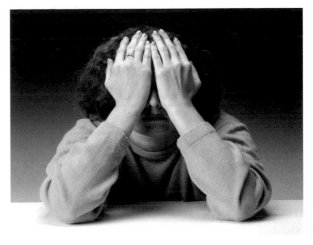

4 Rest your elbows on the table and take a few deep breaths. You will begin to feel your neck muscles relaxing.

5 Let your arms slide apart a little and slowly sink your head into your hands, taking more weight on your elbows. Spend a few moments visualizing a vivid, colorful scene from nature, with changing perspectives.

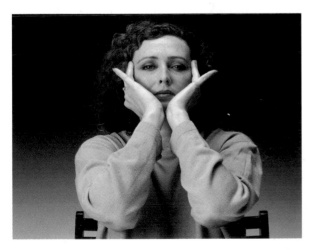

6 After approximately one minute, let the imagery fade and breathe deeply six times. Lightly make contact with the eyeballs by extending your thumb and fingers and flattening your palms over your eye sockets.

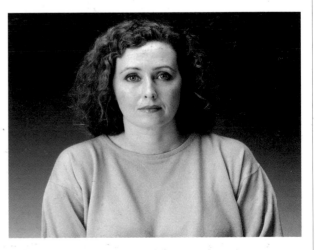

7 Lower your hands to your cheeks and make smooth effleurages from between the eyebrows to the temples, six times.

8 Relax your arms. Widen your eyes for a moment and breathe deeply to conclude the self-massage treatment.

SELF-MASSAGE: FEET

From an early age our feet are confined by shoes in a way that would be unacceptable to any other part of the body. This may result in irreversible compensations such as fallen arches and toe deviations, and freely moving feet are known to provide significant help in preventing heart disease and assisting postoperative circulation. This self-massage can be helpful with headaches, as well as foot discomfort. The water massages are useful when you are suffering from low energy, or just getting back on your feet after an illness.

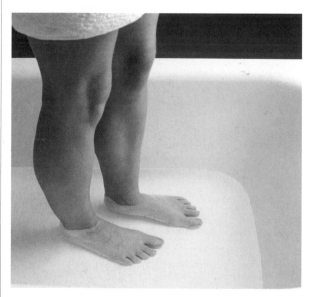

1 Fill a basin with ankle-deep cool water. Take off your shoes and socks and paddle for two minutes, lifting the feet clear of the water.

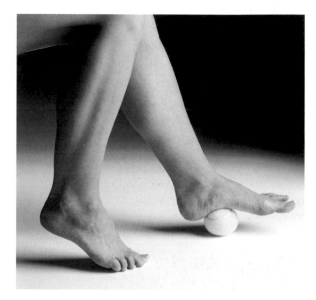

2 Mop your feet dry. Place a ball under one instep and roll the foot backward and forward for one minute. Repeat with the other foot.

3 Walk your feet slowly forward, one foot length at a time, using creeping movements of your toes. Then creep backward.

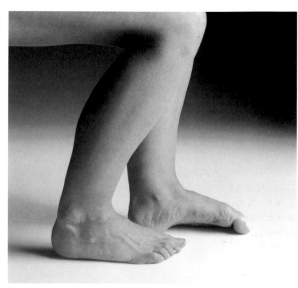

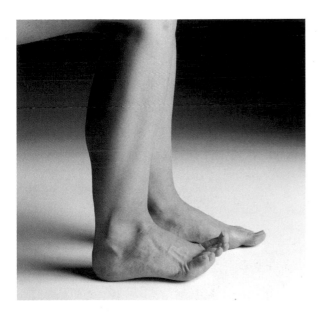

4 Press your left toes onto the floor while drawing your right toes firmly upward, keeping the foot flat. Hold for three seconds, then repeat on the other side.

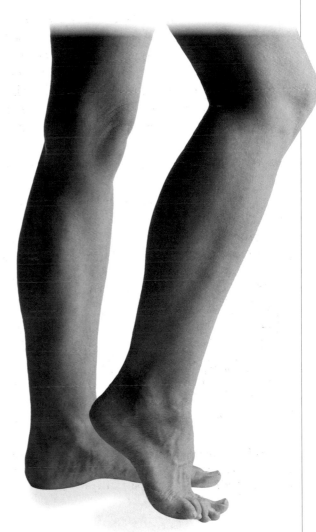

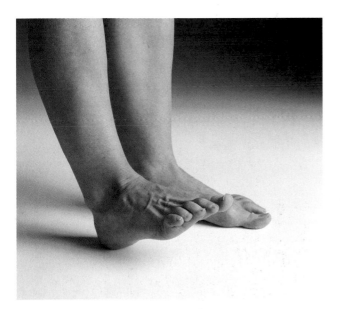

5 While keeping the toes on the ground, bounce the heel of each foot up and down 20 times.

6 Keeping the heels on the ground, bounce the rest of the foot up and down 20 times. Paddle again for one minute, wrap the feet in a towel without drying, and rest with your legs elevated.

SELF-MASSAGE:
INSOMNIA

INSOMNIA APPEARS to be a peculiarly human condition. Even our domesticated animals, who share some of our neurotic traits, do not seem to suffer from sleeplessness. Since one of the biggest differences between human beings and other creatures is brain size, insomnia may be associated with overstimulation of the higher centers. Going to sleep, after all, is not an activity but something that comes over us. This hydrotherapy harmlessly reduces blood flow to the head and helps the brain naturally switch off.

1 If you are unable to fall asleep, then tossing and turning and furiously rubbing your head only succeeds in increasing the blood supply to your brain.

2 Go to the sink and turn on the cold water. Place each wrist under the flow of water for one minute. Your wrists should feel cooled but not chilled.

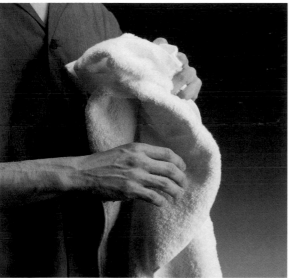

3 Use a towel to mop the water from your hands rather than fully drying them. Then go back to bed.

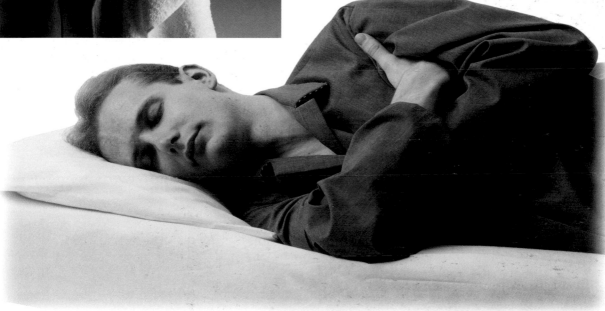

4 Lie on your side so you can insert your hands beneath your underarms. Breathe deeply and assume a sleepy attitude by pretending to be already fast asleep.

5 Almost immediately, you will be aware of increasing warmth in your hands. While this is happening, the blood supply to your brain is reduced. The first time you use this hydrotherapy, you will imagine that you must be dreaming, by which time...

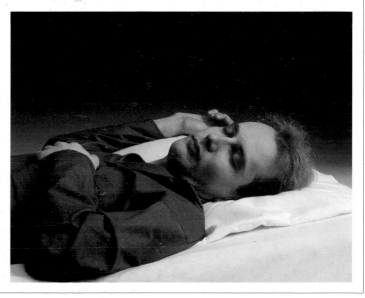

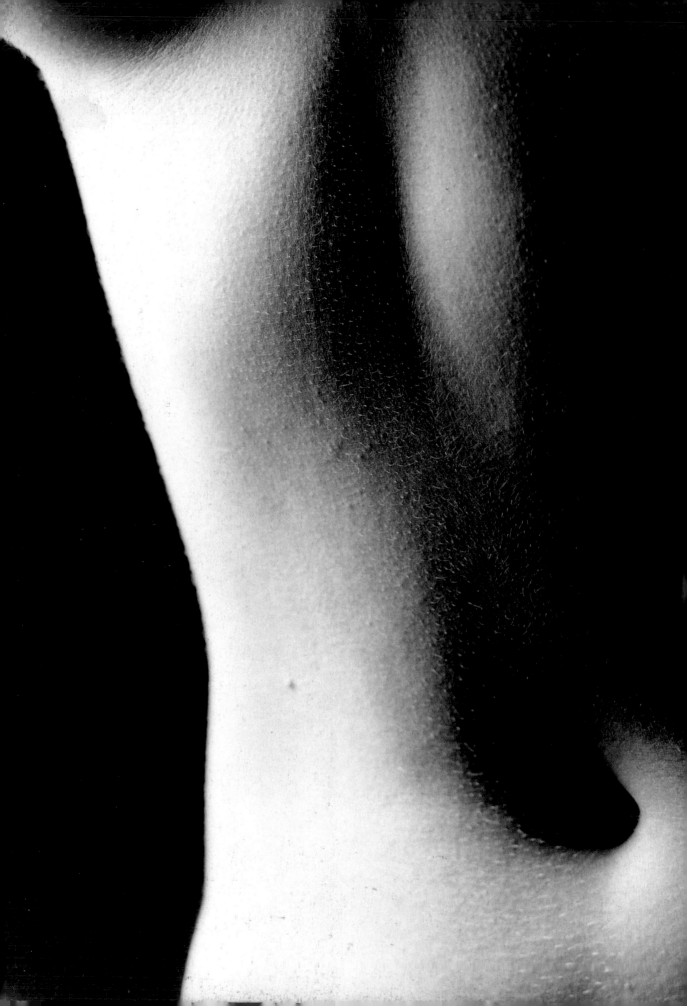

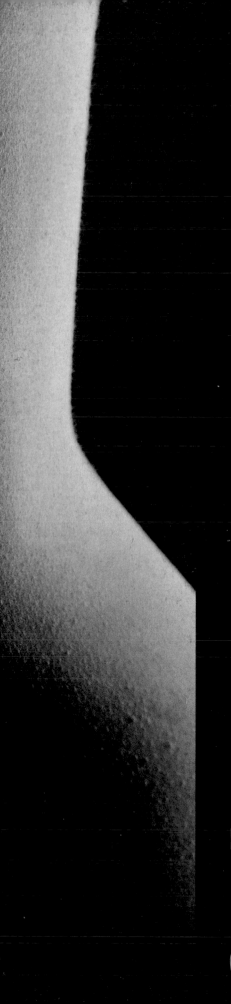

PART EIGHT

MASSAGE AS A PROFESSION

IT IS A MEASURE of the value of massage that many of the benefits described in this book can be provided by enthusiasts who have had only basic instruction. Given a helping and caring disposition, massage skills develop naturally, without the need for complicated theory. Yet successful massage inevitably creates a need for further training, since it tends to attract a wider clientele of family and friends with different expectations, often presenting more complex contraindications to treatment. There is also a greater probability that massage might not be effective, although this will cause disappointment rather than real harm.

ONE WAY OF DEALING with these increasing demands is to convert a casual approach to massage into a profession. This does not always involve abandoning a purely personal interpretation of massage, but it does help channel raw enthusiasm into a disciplined approach that will provide a proper and lasting foundation for future work. The opportunities for providing professional treatment also become broader all the time as more people begin to appreciate the potential of massage. The demand for massage is extending beyond home-based private practice to the workplace, sports center, and even the conventional healthcare center.

Massage students considering professional commitment are often people looking for a subtle

TURNING TO MASSAGE

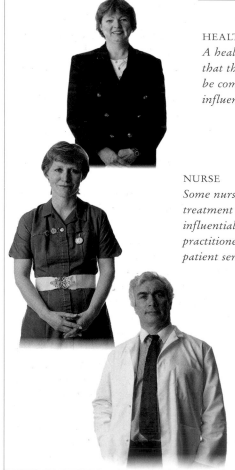

HEALTH WORKER
A health worker may suggest to patients that their conventional healthcare could be complemented by the supportive influence of therapeutic massage.

NURSE
Some nurses, having experienced massage treatment as stress relief, become influential in introducing massage practitioners into community and in-patient services.

PHYSICIANS
Physicians have begun to appreciate that therapeutic massage is not the same as orthodox physiotherapy. This has led to massage becoming integrated into rehabilitation programs for stress-related conditions such as cardiovascular disease.

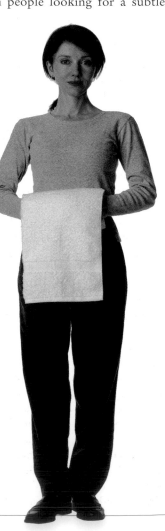

change in career or personal direction. Often, they are mature people who may or may not have a clinical background, but are convinced that massage is the "right" thing to do. Increasingly, however, established professionals from the health field such as nurses, home visitors, and remedial teachers are finding that the supportive influence of massage complements their existing roles. Professional training is absolutely necessary for the established healthcare professional seeking to use massage within work, since it brings his or her level of massage skill up to the high standards necessary to convince skeptical colleagues of its advantages.

MASSAGE TRAINING

There are many routes to becoming a professional, both in outlook and practice. Many organizations offer a formal study of massage, although not all emphasize its humanistic philosophy. Those emphasizing the physiotherapeutic effects of treatments often neglect the emotional benefits of massage. Others who are principally concerned with psychological needs often overlook its obvious mechanical applications. There are also special forms of massage training designed to deal with established medical conditions and diseases. If you are considering professional training, your own interests will determine which course of study you take up.

It is important to identify what is being offered or promised by a training course. It should have clear and realistic objectives, and offer qualifications that are recognized outside its own institution. Massage training is best presented by tutors who are themselves in practice, so they can draw on their own professional experience to help students formulate their plans. The availability of postgraduate supervision will suggest that a training course has confidence in the success of its graduates.

Professionals are encouraged to develop a realistic perspective on their work, which entails self-assessment and external monitoring. Most professional courses include some formal examination system, and students who rely on their instincts find this an unappealing prospect. To achieve accreditation, however, a student should be able to favorably impress an external examiner, who acts as a representative on behalf of future patients. The student should be able to show competence in handling as well as developing expertise, and if the examiner is satisfied, the student will be considered competent to begin professional massage practice.

The many schools of massage operating worldwide use a variety of training methods. Tutorials are usually designed to take account of students' other commitments, so they allow part-time attendance for practical coaching and guidance.

Course lengths vary, but most conform to a system that enables a student to establish a basic practice and increase the variety of therapy available as he or she gains experience.

An example of this approach is the system used by the International Therapy Examination Council (ITEC), an internationally recognized examining body based in Great Britain. ITEC offers a modular examination system that is not affiliated to any particular teaching institution. Students first qualify to become massage practitioners, then work through other complementary therapies like aromatherapy, sports massage, and reflexology to achieve the ultimate qualification of Complementary Therapist. The ITEC system is very flexible and has done much to promote the adoption of massage in healthcare organizations, as well as fostering independent training schools throughout the world.

SETTING UP IN PRACTICE

Successful training is merely the preliminary to professional practice. The word "practice" is used within the profession to emphasize that a practitioner does not begin his or her career "perfected," but uses work experience to transform, develop, and refine the skills learned in training. For some students it can be a daunting transition, bringing feelings of isolation and self-doubt. This is actually a very organic period of development, and many thriving practices are born from the insecurity, frustration, and the creative inspiration of the newly qualified practitioner.

While massage practice is unregulated, many new practitioners will encounter such hesitations sooner or later. Isolation is a significant factor, and new practitioners who join professional organizations, however informal, are less liable to experience such problems. If for any reason it is not possible to keep contact with the training school, or there are no fellow massage practitioners nearby, it is advisable to make friends with other professionals sharing common aims. Practice problems should always be shared and difficult experiences passed on to a trusted listener. Professional stresses are not exclusive to new practitioners, of course, and can be a feature of even the busiest practices.

The decision to transform an interest in massage into a course of formal training should not be taken lightly. Potential practitioners should realize that the rewards of professionalism are in direct proportion to the responsibilities undertaken. This will involve challenge and confrontation, and both physical and intellectual exertion. Developing a professional approach brings great advantages, however, and the increasing popularity of massage offers exciting opportunities for a committed massage therapist.

CASE STUDY 9

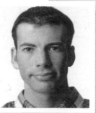

Name: Toby
Age: 23
Personal circumstances: Married

NOTES
• Student at School of Complementary Therapies
• Toby now practices as a sports therapist

TOBY'S INTEREST in massage came from his family background. His parents had regular massage treatments, and Toby remembers being massaged by his mother as a small child. Having been keen on sport, he had also benefited from home massage throughout his schooldays. His contact with massage and sports diminished as he pursued various career interests. Then he made an inspired connection between his earlier enthusiasms and experiences, and decided to train as a sports massage professional.

TOBY CONSULTED a register of massage schools and met the director of a center that specialized in sports massage. The director described the modular syllabus, which provided both theoretical study and practical experience, and Toby signed up.

Toby did well in his training. He found the theoretical aspects of the course satisfied his curiosity about the human body and its potential, and he enjoyed learning remedial skills and the rehabilitation exercises that complement massage. He felt drawn toward studying more about nutrition.

After qualifying, Toby was not fully confident about setting up in practice, so he looked around for a sports center to which he might attach himself, perhaps working alongside an established therapist. This proved difficult, and he had no luck at centers offering general sports facilities. Undaunted, he made another inspired connection. Competitive cycling had been one of his favorite sports in the past, and on the spur of the moment he offered his services to a mountain bike team.

The team manager welcomed Toby's enthusiastic approach and invited him to accompany the team for the World Cup Series – an engagement that took him on tour throughout the United States, Europe, and Canada. The experience he gained was immense, and as he became immersed in the sport he gained a degree of confidence in his therapeutic skills that was to prove invaluable.

Toby's success shows how inspiration and intuition can play an important part in establishing a practice. The transition between being a student and a fully fledged practitioner is fraught with anxiety, and new practitioners tend to forget the leap of faith that, as much as technical achievement, took them to the level of qualification. Toby made that leap again, and his achievements have encouraged him to take further training. He feels confident that his practice can only grow.

CASE STUDY 10

ALTHOUGH MASSAGE WAS not part of her conventional training as a midwife, Lynn became increasingly aware of its benefits through articles published in nursing magazines. The articles reported how massage therapy was being introduced into the care of the elderly, into intensive care rehabilitation, and into the management of pregnancy, and they inspired her to attend an introductory group at a local massage school to experience it for herself.

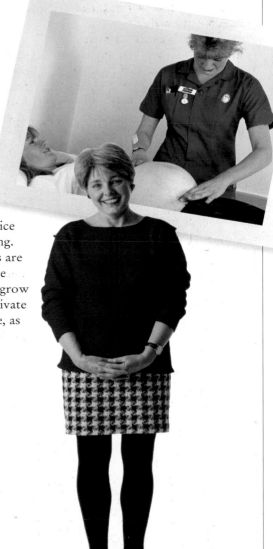

Name: Lynn

Age: 30

Personal circumstances:
Married, one child

NOTES
• Student at School of Complementary Therapies
• Lynn is a professional midwife working within the conventional healthcare system

LYNN ENJOYED THE benefits and stimulation provided by the sessions, and felt that massage could certainly help the women and babies in her care. She was unsure how massage treatment could be integrated into her regular midwifery practice, but despite this she decided to enrol on a professional training course.

Lynn's experiences on the course were a constant source of curiosity to her midwife colleagues, and she massaged several of them in practice for her examinations. When she qualified in both massage and aromatherapy, she felt confident to make a presentation to the team, and during this presentation an idea emerged that was to help establish massage as part of the work of the department. The reasoning was simple: if massage formed part of staff support, it would be easier to present it as a useful aspect of support and care in pregnancy.

Lynn conducted a successful pilot project that included offering simple prenatal and postnatal massage, and guiding partners on birth-assisting massage techniques. The project encouraged other midwives to take up massage training and led to the formation of a massage interest team of midwives that was able to extend the influence of massage throughout all stages of pregnancy. The managers recognized the benefits of massage for midwifery staff, and as the support scheme began to attract more users, it was included into the formal work schedule.

Lynn demonstrated a creative approach to developing a massage practice within a conventional setting. Having found that mothers are reluctant to give up massage treatment as their children grow up, she has established a private practice for continuing care, as well as therapy for women preparing for pregnancy.

USEFUL ADDRESSES

AROMATHERAPY

Australasia

INTERNATIONAL FEDERATION OF
AROMATHERAPISTS
83 Riverdale Road
Hawthorn
Victoria 3122
Australia

Europe

AROMATHERAPY ORGANISATIONS
COUNCIL
3 Latimer Close
Braybrooke
Market Harborough
Leicester LE16 8LN

INTERNATIONAL FEDERATION
OF AROMATHERAPISTS
Stamford House
2–4 Chiswick High Road
London W4 1TH
Great Britain
Tel: 44 181 742 2605
Fax: 44 181 742 2606

INTERNATIONAL SOCIETY OF
PROFESSIONAL AROMATHERAPISTS
ISPA House
82 Ashby Road
Hinckley
Leics OE10 1SN
Great Britain
Tel: 44 1455 637987
Fax: 44 1455 890956

North America

AMERICAN ALLIANCE OF AROMA
THERAPY
PO Box 750428
Petaluma
California 94975-0428
USA
Tel: 1 707 778 6762
Fax: 1 707 769 0868

AMERICAN AROMATHERAPY
ASSOCIATION
PO Box 3679
South Pasadena
California 91031
USA
Tel: 818 457 1742

NATIONAL ASSOCIATION OF HOLISTIC
AROMATHERAPY
PO Box 17622
Boulder
Colorado 80308-0622
USA
Tel: 1 303 258 3791

AYURVEDIC FOOT PRESSURE MASSAGE

Europe

DEVON SCHOOL OF YOGA
Fourways
Stevens Cross
Sidford
Devon EX10 9QL

HYDROTHERAPY

Europe

UK COLLEGE OF HYDROTHERAPY
515 Hagley Road
Birmingham B66 4AX
Great Britain
Tel: 44 121 429 9191
Fax: 44 121 478 0871

North America

AQUATIC EXERCISE ASSOCIATION
PO Box 1609
Nokomis
Florida 34274
USA
Tel: 1 813 486 8600

INVERSION THERAPY

Europe

SCHOOL OF COMPLEMENTARY THERAPIES
38 South Street
Exeter EX1 1ED
Great Britain

MASSAGE

Australasia

ASSOCIATION OF MASSAGE THERAPISTS
3/33 Denham Street
Bondai
New South Wales NSW 2026
Australia

NEW ZEALAND ASSOCIATION OF
THERAPEUTIC MASSAGE PRACTITIONERS
PO Box 375
Hamilton
New Zealand

Europe

MASSAGE THERAPY INSTITUTE OF
GREAT BRITAIN
PO Box 276
London NW2 4NR
Great Britain

SCHOOL OF COMPLEMENTARY THERAPIES
38 South Street
Exeter EX1 1ED
Great Britain

INTERNATIONAL THERAPY
EXAMINATION COUNCIL
James House
Oakelbrook Mill
Newent
Gloucestershire GL15 1HD
Great Britain
Tel: 44 1531 821875

MASSAGE TRAINING INSTITUTE
24 Highbury Road
London
Great Britain
Tel: 44 171 226 5313

NORTHERN INSTITUTE
100 Waterloo Road
Blackpool
Lancashire FY4 1AW
Great Britain
Tel: 44 1253 403548

North America

AMERICAN MASSAGE
THERAPY ASSOCIATION
820 Davis Street
Suite 100
Evanston
Illinois 60201-4444
USA
Tel: 1 708 864 0123
Fax: 1 708 864 1178

INTERNATIONAL ASSOCIATION
OF INFANT MASSAGE
PO Box 438
Elma
New York 14059-0438
USA
Tel: 1 716 652 9789
Fax: 1 716 652 1990

INTERNATIONAL MASSAGE ASSOCIATION
3000 Connecticut Avenue NW
Apt 102
Washington, DC 20008
USA
Tel: 1 202 387 6555
Fax: 1 202 332 0531

NATIONAL ASSOCIATION
OF MASSAGE THERAPY
PO Box 1400
Westminster
Colorado 80030-1400
USA
Tel: 1 800 776 6268

ON-SITE THERAPY
(SEATED MASSAGE)

Europe

SCHOOL OF COMPLEMENTARY THERAPIES
38 South Street
Exeter EX1 1ED
Great Britain

OSTEOPATHY

Australasia

CHIROPRACTORS AND OSTEOPATHS'
REGISTRATION BOARD OF VICTORIA
PO Box 59
Carlton South
Victoria 3053
Australia
Tel: 61 3 349 3000
Fax: 61 3 349 3003

NSW CHIROPRACTORS AND
OSTEOPATHIC REGISTRATION BOARD
PO Box K599
Haymarket
New South Wales 2000
Australia
Tel: 61 2 281 0884
Fax: 61 2 281 2030

Europe

GENERAL REGISTER AND COUNCIL
OF OSTEOPATHS
56 London Street
Reading
Berks RG1 4SQ
Great Britain
Tel: 44 1734 576585
Fax: 44 1734 566246

North America

AMERICAN ACADEMY OF OSTEOPATHY
3500 DePauw Boulevard
Suite 1080
Indianapolis
Indiana 46268-139
USA
Tel: 1 317 879 1881
Fax: 1 317 879 0563

AMERICAN OSTEOPATHIC ASSOCIATION
142 East Ohio Street
Chicago
Illinois 60611
USA
Tel: 1 312 280 5800
Fax: 1 312 280 3860

POLARITY THERAPY

Europe

UK POLARITY THERAPY ASSOCIATION
Monomark House
27 Old Gloucester Street
London WC1N 3XX
Great Britain
Tel: 44 1483 417714

North America

AMERICAN POLARITY THERAPY ASSOC.
2888 Bluff Street
Suite 149
Boulder
Colorado 80301 USA
Tel: 1 303 545 2080
Fax: 1 303 545 2161

REFLEXOLOGY

Asia

CHINESE SOCIETY OF REFLEXOLOGISTS
Xuanwu Hospital
Capital Institute of Medicine
Chang Chun Street
Beijing
China

RWO-SHR HEALTH INSTITUTE
INTERNATIONAL
1–11 Wilayah Shopping Centre
Jalan Campbell 50100
Kuala Lumpur
Malaysia

Australasia

NEW ZEALAND REFLEXOLOGY
ASSOCIATION
PO Box 31 084
Auckland 4
New Zealand

REFLEXOLOGY ASSOCIATION
OF AUSTRALIA
15 Kedumba Crescent
Turramurra 2074
New South Wales
Australia

Europe

ASSOCIATION OF REFLEXOLOGISTS
27 Old Gloucester Street
London WC1N 3XX
Great Britain
Tel: 44 990 673320

ASSOCIATION OF
VACUFLEX REFLEXOLOGY
PO Box 93
Tadworth
Surrey KT20 7YB
Great Britain
Tel/Fax: 44 1737 842961

FEDERATION OF PRECISION
REFLEXOLOGISTS
38 South Street
Exeter EX1 1ED
Great Britain

INTERNATIONAL INSTITUTE
OF REFLEXOLOGY
15 Hartfield Close
Tonbridge
Kent
Great Britain
Tel/Fax: 44 1732 350629

North America

ASSOCIATION OF VACUFLEX
REFLEXOLOGY
1951 Glenarie Avenue
North Vancouver V7P 1XP
Canada
Tel: 1 604 986 7121

ASSOCIATION OF VACUFLEX
REFLEXOLOGY
2222 Kilkare Parkway
Pt Pleasant
New Jersey 08742
USA
Tel: 1 908 892 7566

INTERNATIONAL INSTITUTE OF
REFLEXOLOGY
PO Box 12642
Saint Petersberg
Florida 33733
USA
Tel: 1 813 343 4811

REFLEXOLOGY ASSOCIATION OF
AMERICA
4012 S. Rainbow Boulevard
Box K585
Las Vegas
Nevada 89103-2509
USA

REFLEXOLOGY ASSOCIATION OF CANADA
(RAC)
11 Glen Cameron Road
Unit 4
Thornhill
Ontario L8T 4NB
Canada
Tel: 1 905 889 5900

SHIATSU

Europe

THE SHIATSU SOCIETY
5 Foxcote
Wokingham
Berkshire RG11 3PG
Great Britain

FURTHER READING

(All books on this list have been published in the UK, unless otherwise noted)

AROMATHERAPY

Aromatherapy for Healing the Spirit
by Gabrielle Mojay
(Gaia, 1996)

Aromatherapy for Pregnancy and Childbirth
by Margaret Fawcett
(Element Books, 1993)

Aromatherapy from Provence
by Nelly Grosjean
(C.W. Daniel, 1994)

Aromatherapy: Massage with Essential Oils
by Christine Wildwood
(Element Books, 1991)

Complete Aromatherapy Handbook
by Susanne Fischer-Rizzi
(Stirling, 1990, USA)

Massage and Aromatherapy
by Andrew Vickers
(Chapman & Hall, 1996)

AYURVEDIC

Ancient Indian Massage
by Harish Johari
(Munshiram Manoharial, 1984)

GENERAL

Beard's Massage by Wood & Becker
(3rd Edition, W.B. Saunders, 1964)

Massage: A Practical Introduction
by Stewart Mitchell
(Element Books, 1992)

Mosby's Fundamentals of Therapeutic Massage
by Sandy Fritz
(Mosby Lifeline, 1995)

The Complete Book of Massage
Clare Maxwell-Hudson
(Dorling Kindersley, 1988)

Tidy's Massage and Remedial Exercises 11th ed.
(John Wright & Son, 1968)

Bodywatching
by Desmond Morris
(Jonathan Cape, 1986)

Bodyline
by Arthur Balaskus
(Sidgwick & Jackson, 1977)

Manipulation and Mobilisation
by Susan L. Edmund
(Mosby, 1993)

Principles of Anatomy and Physiology
by Tortora & Grabowski
(Harper Collins, 1996)

Principles and Practices of Physical Therapy
by W. Arnould-Taylor
(Stanley Thornes, 1997)

Some Body!
by Pete Rowan
(Riverswift, 1994)

Superfoods
by Michael Van Stratten & Barbara Griggs
(Dorling Kindersley, 1993)

The Bassett Atlas of Human Anatomy
by Robert A. Chase
(Benjamin Cummings, 1989)

Touch – An Exploration
by N. Autton
(Longman & Todd, 1989)

The New Atlas of the Human Body
by Vannini and Pogliano, translated by R. Jolly
(Chancellor Press, 1980)

Visualising Muscles
by John Cody
(Kansas University Press, 1990, USA)

HYDROTHERAPY

The Complete Book of Water Therapy
by Dian Dinsin Buchman
(Keats, 1994)

Water and Nature Cure
by C. Leslie Thomson
(Kingston Clinic, Edinburgh, 1955)

Water Babies
by Erik Sidenbladh
(A and C Black, 1983)

Water and Sexuality
by Michel Odent
(Arkana, 1990)

REFLEXOLOGY

*The Complete Illustrated Guide
to Reflexology*
by Inge Dougans
(Element Books, UK/US, 1996)

*The Reflexology and Colour
Therapy Workbook*
by Pauline Wills
(Element Books, 1992)

Reflexology – The Ancient Answer
by Ann Gilanders
(Jenny Lee Publishing, 1994)

The Reflexology Partnership
by Adamson and Harris
(Kyle Cathie, 1995)

Zone Therapy Using Foot Massage
by Astrid Goosman-Legger
(C.W. Daniel, 1983)

SHIATSU

The Book of Shiatsu
by P. Lundberg
(Gaia Books, 1992)

Shiatsu: The Complete Guide
by C. Jarmey and G. Mojay
(Thorsons, 1991)

*Shiatsu: Japanese Massage for Health
and Fitness*
by Elaine Liechti
(Element Books, 1992)

The Shiatsu Workbook
by N. Dawes
(Piatkus Books, 1991)

SPORTS

Athletic Ability and the Anatomy of Motion
by Rolf Wirhed
(Wolfe Medical, 1984)

Sport and Remedial Massage Therapy
by Mel Cash
(Ebury Press, 1996)

Stretching Without Pain
by W. Paul Blakey
(Bibliotek Books, 1994)

The Colour Atlas of Injury and Sport
by JGP Williams
(Wolfe, 1990)

JOURNALS

East-West Natural Health
17 Station Street, Box 1200, Brookline Village,
MA 02147 (USA)

Massage Magazine
1315 W. Mallon, Spokane WA 99201 (USA)

Natural Therapies Database UK
47 Ashby Avenue, Chessington, Surrey KT9 2BT

Peak Performance
67-71 Goswell Road, London EC1V 7EN

The Institute of Health Sciences Journal
PO Box 457, London NW2 4BR

The International Journal of Aromatherapy
PO Box 746, Hove, E. Sussex BN3 3XA

GLOSSARY

Abduct: anatomical term meaning to move (a limb) away from the middle line.

Adduct: opposite of the above: to move toward the middle.

Anatomy: the science of the shape and structure of the body and its parts. Initially daunting for serious massage students, they have the advantage of learning the living anatomy of partners as they learn to massage.

Artery: a tube-like vessel that carries blood away from the heart to the rest of the body. Arteries become progressively smaller, becoming *arterioles*, then minute *capillaries*, only one cell in diameter. Research has shown that stressful Western lifestyle can cause arteries to degenerate prematurely.

Arthritis: inflammation of the structures within a skeletal joint (*rheumatoid arthritis*). When the lining of the bones which form a joint become worn and painful this is called *osteoarthritis*.

Autonomic Nervous System: explains how the involuntary or unconscious functions, like breathing and digestion, are controlled. The ANS has two complementary aspects: *sympathetic* nerves, concerned with stimulating, energetic action (speeding up); and *parasympathetic* nerves, which inhibit (slow down). Through these mechanisms the body's internal environment is kept in harmony.

Bronchi: the branch-like windpipe which reaches into the lungs, continually subdividing in the manner of a tree. The smaller bronchi are called *bronchioles* and terminate in "buds," *alveoli*, at which point the respiratory gases exchange. While the "trees" of our lungs breathe out carbon dioxide, the trees on earth breathe it in; their out-breathing of oxygen is taken up by our lungs.

Bursa: fluid-filled pads which help protect the joints of the limbs. When a joint is subjected to repeated, excessive pressures from without, the bursa may become inflamed: *bursitis*.

Biceps: a muscle which has two points of attachment to a bone (lit. "two heads"), e.g. the calf muscle, which can be felt behind the knee. Three points give *Triceps*, at the back of the upper arm: four points for *Quadriceps*, on the front of the thigh.

Caudal: toward the tail (of the spine).

Central Nervous System: the actions of the nerves of the body which comprise the brain, spinal cord and peripheries. The CNS is characterized as controlling the conscious and deliberate movements of muscle and mind. *Motor* nerves relay instructions to the muscles to contract: *sensor* nerves record pain, heat, cold, etc. for the brain's interpretation. Nerves exit from spaces between the joints of the vertebral column and can be adversely affected by disorders of the joint.

Cephalic: toward the head.

Circulatory System: the movement of the blood around the body via the heart and its vessels, arteries and veins, and the lymphatics.

Couch: a custom-built table for massage treatment. It may be fixed or portable and should be designed to the appropriate height for the practitioner. (To test: stand sideways by the couch, arms by your side; flex your wrist so that your palm is now horizontal – this is the recommended couch height for you.)

Diagnosis: recognition of which disease a person has. Can lead to categorization and depersonalization of the patient/client. Some physicians prefer to ask: "Which type of person has this disease?"

Diaphragm: the dome-like muscle which separates the contents of the chest from the abdomen. The diaphragm's active function is to assist full working of the lungs, while rhythmically massaging the digestive organs.

Dermis: the true skin, lying just beneath the outermost protective layer. The skin retains delicate sensitivity while forming an effective waterproof and thermal barrier for the body.

Dorsal: toward the back.

Endocrine System: describes the influence of hormones on the body. Hormones are chemical messengers, concentrated in glands strategically placed around the body. At critical times in our development, hormones are released directly into the blood stream to bring about subtle changes in functioning.

Eversion: to turn outward.

Fibrositis: inflammation of the covering of the muscles, arising from excess tension or injury.

G5: a mechanical massage appliance. It is hand-held and does not substitute but can complement hand massage. Also useful in treating injuries, the G5 has the basic design of a circular head of rubber which vibrates horizontally.

Hypertension: abnormal and undesirably high blood pressure. Can be evaluated subjectively or by the *sphygomanometer*, an inflatable cuff placed around the arm. Although the sphygomanometer translates simply to mean "to measure the pressure," its appearance and mere attachment to the arm often significantly raises the blood pressure!

Hypotension: low blood pressure. Low blood pressure is not regarded as particularly unhealthy in the U.K. (although it is in Germany, where hypotensives are medicated in the same manner as hypertensives in the U.K.). lower than average blood pressure is accepted as less strenuous for the body, but higher-pressure personalities naturally question what the slower moving hypotensives are conserving themselves *for*!

Immobilization: placing the body in such a position so as to minimize strain, especially if injured. *Examples:* resting a flexed knee over a pillow; placing the arm in a sling.

Insertion: the end of a muscle which is attached to the bone it intends to move. *Example:* the main calf muscle *Gastrocnemius* inserts on to the heel bone and by pulling on it, points the foot.

Inversion: to turn outside in.

Kyphosis: derangement of the spinal column resulting in an exaggerated outward curve in the thoracic spine.

Lordosis: excessive inward curvature of the spinal column at the lumbar vertebrae.

Lymphatic System: a complementary circulation which parallels the venous return. Lymph, which is the water drained from tissues, together with disinfecting white blood cells, washes through from the peripheral body, cleansing and tidying *en route* back to the upper chest where it returns to the whole blood just before entry to the heart. The lymph is periodically drained as it passes through *nodes*, conveniently placed in crevices of the body: behind the knee, in the groin, under the arms, etc. The nodes also contain extra-powerful cleansing cells, *lymphocytes*, which can be transferred to the lymph in transit for emergencies of accident or illness.

Massage: manipulation of the soft tissues of the body for therapeutic purposes. Records of forms of message have been found in all cultures from the earliest times.

Medial: toward the center.

Partner: someone who agrees to be massaged or exchange massage.

Posture: efficient alignment of the skeleton relative to any position but usually associated with upright stance. Posture can also mean attitude, which suggests that positioning has emotional and physical components.

Practitioner: one who gives massage professionally or with a committed interest.

Prone: facing downward.

Psychology: the study of thought, emotion and behavior, distinct from *psychiatry*, which is a medical speciality which treats diseases of the mind.

Quadriceps: see **Biceps**.

Reflex: involuntary contraction of a muscle resulting from an unexpected stimulus. Occurs as in the "tickling" mistake of a massage stroke which is too sudden or deep.

Rheumatism: name formerly used for general forms of arthritis.

Sciatica: inflammation of the sciatic nerve, which runs from the lower back, behind the leg all the way underneath the foot. Sciatica often accompanies disorders of the vertebrae when these are misaligned or compressed.

Scoliosis: lateral (sideways) deviation of the spine, which, viewed from behind, creates "S" shaped curves. The three common spinal deviations described in the glossary may be *congenital* (since birth), or as a result of injury or adaptation to environment.

Slipped Disc: a misnomer for a pressurized intervertebral disc (usually lumbar). The disc, which is made up of a cushion-like material, cannot actually slip but sometimes protrudes and interferes with the nerves exiting the spine. Discs are not "put back in" even by the most exotic techniques, but are released by support and gentle traction.

Specialist: a practitioner with a concentrated approach, usually well experienced but in danger of "finding out more and more about less and less."

Stress: an excessive, unrelieved cycle of tension. Distinct from *strain*, which is self-regulating (something is hurting and we usually "stop"), stress may be harder to recognize subjectively.

Supine: facing upward.

Tendon: the fibers at a muscle's end which attach it to a bone. Overuse of a muscle may inflame the tendon, producing *tendonitis*.

Therapy: literally "to care for" and accompany a person in their illness. Parallel of *patient* ("receptive to healing").

Tonus: slight, continuous contraction of muscles, which maintains posture and helps blood flow. Listening into tonus with our ear against the skin, we would hear crackling tensions, similar to sounds heard during head-rolling exercises.

Traction: lengthening of the spine, usually from external stretch. Spontaneous traction occurs throughout the spine on each exhalation.

Trauma: literally "wound", having physical and psychological consequences.

Treatment: what the therapist offers: a "treat."

Triceps: See **Biceps**.

Vasoconstriction: diminution of the smaller arteries; pallor, the effect of cold water on the skin's blood vessels.

Vasodilatation: expansion of the smaller arteries; blushing; the effect of alcohol on the skin's blood vessels (we feel "warm"). The rapidly alternating vasoconstriction and vasodilation of the abdomen's tiny blood vessels when we are nervous gives the sensation of "butterflies."

Vein: a tube-like vessel which conducts blood back to the heart. Relatively superficial, the veins can be seen and felt, especially when *varicose*, full of pressure and struggling to overcome the effects of gravity.

INDEX